Surgery of Stapes Fixations

Istvan Sziklai
Editor

Surgery of Stapes Fixations

Springer

Editor
Istvan Sziklai
Department of Otorhinolaryngology
University of Debrecen
Debrecen
Hungary

ISBN 978-3-319-28574-0 ISBN 978-3-319-28576-4 (eBook)
DOI 10.1007/978-3-319-28576-4

Library of Congress Control Number: 2016935717

Springer Cham Heidelberg New York Dordrecht London

Printed on acid-free paper

Springer International Publishing AG Switzerland is part of Springer Science+Business Media (www.springer.com)

Preface

Conductive hearing loss due to immobility of the stapes was considered as otosclerosis from the beginning of the history of otology. Still today many ear surgeons think that hearing loss related to stapes fixation is otosclerotic in origin. This *dogma* is attempted to elucidate in this book since gradually increasing evidences of non-otosclerotic stapes fixation and its relatively high incidence are accumulated. The etiology of stapes fixation influences the surgical technique to be chosen. A new horizon of preoperative diagnosis of otosclerosis is opened by the observation that measles virus particles in the otosclerotic footplate are all the time present in otosclerosis and that antimeasles IgG concentration in the sera of patients with otosclerosis-related conductive hearing loss is low as if the immune system of these patients wouldn't recognize the vaccination. Different new surgical solutions are introduced in stapes surgery, i.e., laser fenestration of stapes and endoscopic approach of the oval window niche. Robotic surgery of the stapes is still experimental; however, it can be predicted that in the near future robotic procedures will be included in the *repertoire* of the surgery of stapes fixations. Manufacturing piston prosthesis for reconstruction of the ossicular chain after stapedectomy/stapedotomy followed a greatful evolution as to shape, material, and crimping technology. The good hearing outcome after surgery of stapes fixation makes this otologic procedure the most effective tool for hearing reconstruction.

Stapes operation can be combined with implantation of active middle ear implants for amplification of sound-evoked vibrations in the cochlea when mild sensorineural component of a mixed hearing loss indicate it. Quality of sound sensation is better by these devices than those provided by conventional or open-fit hearing aids. This can improve the satisfaction and the quality of life of the patients. Far advanced otosclerosis with moderate to severe sensorineural hearing loss is an indication for cochlear implantation. These patients are postlingually deafened individuals and consequently their hearing rehabilitation by the implant is very successful.

Good surgical techniques, devices, prostheses, and patient care still cannot provide with 100 % success rate in hearing results. Today the standard hearing improvement after stapes surgery is closure of the air-bone gap to 10 dB or less. Preoperative imaging before stapedectomy/stapedotomy is essential to clarify potential hazards given by anatomical abnormalities. Stapes surgery is safe, but still in spite of rigorous rules followed, a 1 % failure rate is calculated. Major and minor failures teach us to respect the versatility of human anatomy and physiology.

All above aspects of stapes surgery are considered in this book. The authors of different chapters are well known and internationally recognized representatives in the field. Thanking them their contribution, I hope we provide a useful textbook for those interested in the topic.

Debrecen, Hungary Istvan Sziklai

Contents

List of Videos

Video 4.1 Scutoplasty. Small piece of the scutum is separated by a chisel in a left ear. The skin of the external auditory meatus is already dislocated anteriorly; the fibrocartilaginous annulus of the drum is elevated. Behind it the middle ear cavity is opened. The chiseled bone fragment is dislocated by a needle. Care is taken to separate the chorda tympani from it. The bone fragment is removed by a forceps and the incudostapedial joint comes into viewfield

Video 4.2 Mobility of the ossicular chain. The incudostapedial joint is exposed in a left ear. The malleus is moved by a needle to check its mobility. The lenticular process moves well, but the stapes is fixed. The oval window niche is highly vascularized which is supportive for otosclerosis

Video 4.3 Stapedectomy when the whole stapes can be removed. The incudostapedial joint is disarticulated after fenestration of the footplate by a needle in a left ear. The chorda tympani is preserved. Small movements of the superstructure may help to separate the footplate from the oval window. This can be successful in non-otosclerotic stapes fixations usually. The whole stapes is then removed by a hook. Shea cup piston of 4.75 mm length is inserted to connect the incus to the vestibule. This prosthesis is a self-crimping type

Video 4.4 Hemostasis in the stapedial niche. To obtain bloodless surgical field in the oval window niche, epinephrine soaked gelfoam balls are placed onto the long process of the incus and into the niche before fenestration of the footplate

Video 4.5 Fenestration of the footplate. The footplate is fenestrated by a needle in the posterior one-third of the footplate before disarticulation in a left ear. Fenestration should be performed with small force in non-otosclerotic cases like this one because the bone is very thin in the middle of the footplate

Video 4.6 Stapedectomy when the superstructure and the footplate is removed in pieces (left ear). (**a**) The superstructure breaks down from the footplate when an attempt is made to remove the stapes. The hole made prior to disarticulation of the incudostapedial joint can be seen in the footplate. (**b**) The posterior half of the

1 Some Pioneers in Early Stapes Surgery

R.A. Tange

Otosclerosis is an affection of the middle and the inner ear. The stapes plays an important role in this affection. It was Giovanni Ingrassia (1510–1580) who by accident discovered the stapes in the middle ear during cadaver studies. The physiology of the hearing organ was described for the first time by Volcher Koyter (1534–1600). Hieronymus Capivacci (†1589) found a test to distinguish between perceptive and conducting hearing loss. It was Antonio Valsalva (1666–1723) who recognized the nature of the disease nowadays called otosclerosis. In his *De aure humana tractatus*, written while he was Professor of Anatomy at Bologna, he was the first to connect deafness during life with an ossified and fixed stapes found at autopsy. Valsalva gave the earliest description of the pathological otosclerotic process. Giovanni Morgagni (1761) refined the anatomical and pathological studies on the middle ear of his teacher Valsalva. Meckel (1771) and Domenico Cotugno demonstrated that there was fluid and no air inside the labyrinth. Joseph Toynbee of London (1815–1866) focused attention upon the connection between stapes ankylosis and deafness after his study of 1,659 human temporal bones in 1841. He found that in no less than 136 out of 1,149 dissected temporal bones, stapes ankylosis could be demonstrated. He distinguished four pathologic variations of stapes fixation [1]. One of the first observations of an otosclerotic focus at the stapes footplate was by Adam Politzer in 1862 (Fig. 1.1). He described a case of white bony formation at the place of an immobile stapes footplate in a cadaver.

Politzer could not explain the etiology of the process leading to the new bone formation and fixation of the stapes in human temporal bones. Because of the lack of signs of infection around the stapes in his histological slides, he stated that the ankylosis of the stapes could not be regarded as a result of middle ear infections. Von Troltsch (1881) used the term "sclerosis" for stapes fixation. He thought that sclerosis of the tympanic cavity mucosa caused stapes fixation. It was in 1890 that L. Katz from Ludwighaven gave a first full pathological report together with the results of the clinical examination of the patient with otosclerosis and finally filled in the completed clinical picture of the disease. He found microscopic evidence of otosclerosis resulting in stapes fixation. In 1893, Politzer described otosclerosis as a clinical entity and further characterized its pathology as a "Primary Disease of the Bony Labyrinthine Capsule," in which neoplastic bone gradually takes the place of normal bone and produces ankylosis of the stapes. With the early recognition that the otosclerostic process was in fact an immobilizing of the stapes in the oval window, many treatments were used experimentally without a full clinical appreciation of the actual process.

R.A. Tange
Department of ORL, UMCU, University of Utrecht, PO box 85500, Utrecht 3508 GA, The Netherlands
e-mail: r.a.tange@umcutrecht.nl

I. Sziklai (ed.), *Surgery of Stapes Fixations*, DOI 10.1007/978-3-319-28576-4_1

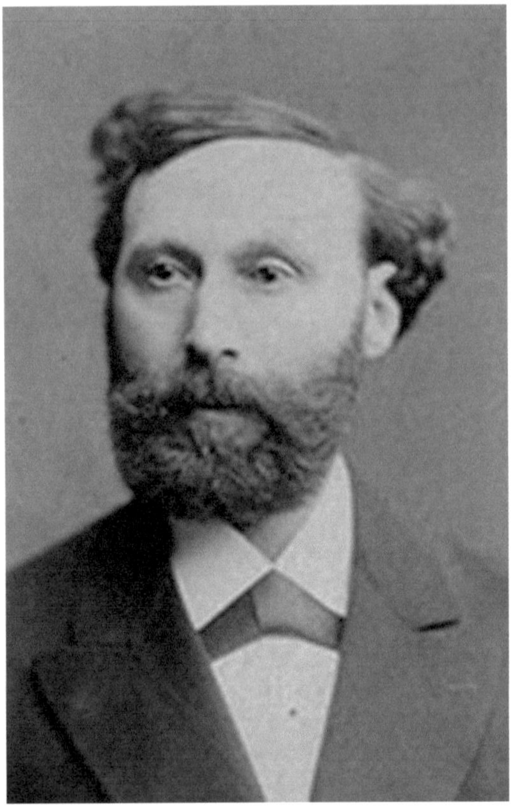

Fig. 1.1 Adam Politzer

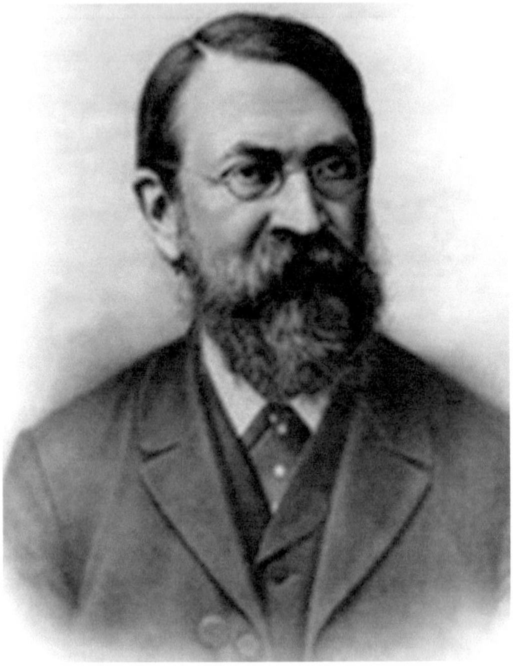

Fig. 1.2 Ernst Mach

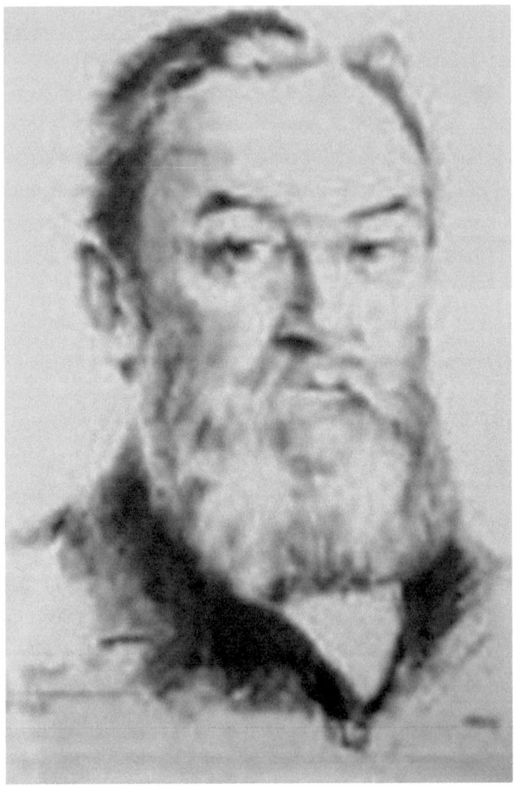

Fig. 1.3 Johannes Kessel

Because of the failure of these conservative methods, surgical intervention for the problem became an option. Ernst Mach (1838–1916; Fig. 1.2) from Prague was the first to perform experimental mobilization of the stapes with Johannes Kessel.

After experimental operations on dog and pigeon, Kessel (1839–1907; Fig. 1.3) performed his stapes mobilization and extraction operation in 1876. The problem of the mobilization of the stapes was the approach straight through the tympanic membrane. Kessel decided to go directly to the stapes footplate after ablation of the membrane and the middle ear ossicles after an antroatticotomy. Because in many cases the results were not satisfactory, Kessel also extracted the stapes. Ear surgery at that time was not without danger. There were no microscopes or antibiotics available, which meant that there was a great risk of – often fatal – meningitis. Furthermore, a facial-nerve palsy and intensive bleeding could occur. In 1876,

J. Michel from Grenoble also published his experience with the mobilization. E. Boucheron from Paris published in 1888 60 cases of stapes mobilization with a success lasting more than 16 months. Unfortunately, there were frequent infections in most of the cases. Boucheron was some kind of prophet when he wrote about the stapes mobilization: "C'est une opération d'avenir. Il faudra, comme l'opération de la cataracte, attendre cent ans pour en apprécier la valeur." Miot from Paris reported in 1896 on 126 cases of mobilization of the stapes, 24 cases of which were otosclerosis. In 18 of the 24 cases, a good result was demonstrated. In the USA, C.J. Blake (1843–1919) (Fig 1.4) and F.L. Jack (1861–1951) (Fig. 1.5) from Boston and J.H. Burnett from Philadelphia reported remarkable improvement in hearing after removal of the stapes. The results were not long-lasting. In only a few cases, the result remained stable after 10 years after the surgery (Table 1.1).

The surgical approach to the fixated stapes in otosclerosis was unsuccessful due to recurrent infections and the risk of intracranial abscesses. To avoid the actual focus of disease, K.A. Passow (1859–1926) (Fig. 1.6) from Heidelberg made in 1897 an opening to the cochlea in the medial wall of the middle ear close to the oval window. The promontory was trephined and the opening covered with a mucoperiosteal flap. This can be considered as the first cochleostomy ever. No lasting improvement was obtained, and often the hearing was made worse.

H.A. Alderton (1896) from New York tried to drill with a dental drill through the stapes footplate to create a fistula, but the results of this procedure were without lasting success. B. Floderus from Denmark in 1898 and C.A. Ballance (1856–1936) in 1900 were the first suggesting the creating of a fistula into the horizontal semicircular canal to stop vertigo problems and in some cases to improve hearing. By accident, Ballance opened the horizontal semicircular canal during mastoid surgery. He covered the fistula by a thin layer of squamous epithelium skin transplant and observed that the preoperative vertigo was diminished and the hearing improved. Recurrent infections were an important reason that these fistulae operations for otosclerosis were unsuccessful.

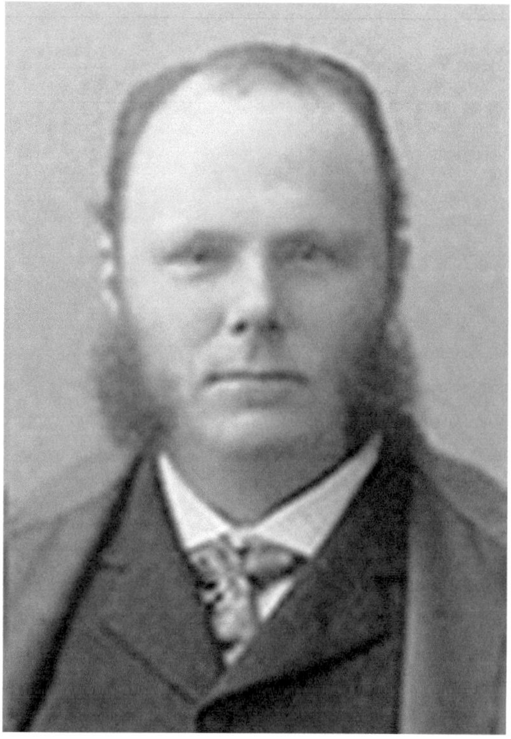

Fig, 1.4 Clarence Blake

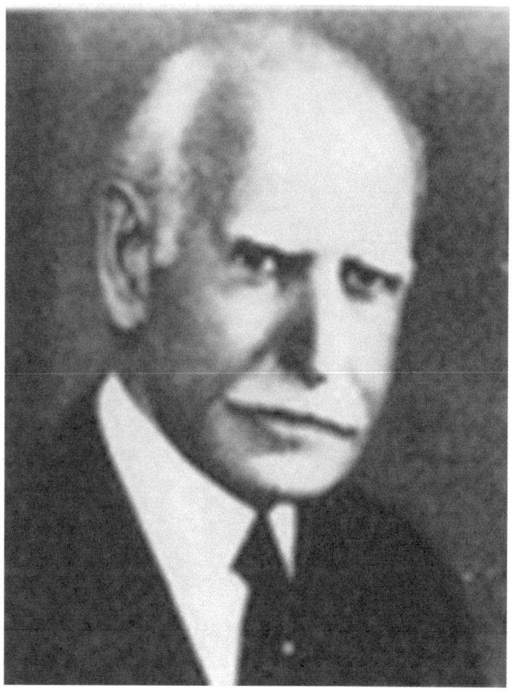

Fig. 1.5 Frederick Jack

Table 1.1 Some of the well-known pioneers of otosclerosis surgery in the nineteenth century [1]

Surgeon	Year	Place	Result
Mach	1870	Prague	First experimental mobilization of the stapes
Kessel	1876	Jena	Mobilization of the stapes
Michel	1876	Grenoble	Mobilization of the stapes
Lucae	1884	Berlin	Repeated percussion of the chain
Boucheron	1888	Paris	60 cases, good results/frequent infections
Gellée	1888	Paris	Blind mobilization through membrane
Sexton	1889	New York	Removal of the stapes
Schwartze	1890	Halle	42 % success
Blake	1890	Boston	Good results but not long-lasting
Jack	1892	Boston	Good results but not long-lasting
Miot	1896	Paris	24/18 = 75 % success
Alderton	1896	New York	Footplate perforation with dental drill
Floderus	1899	Denmark	Fistula in semicircular canal
Faraci	1899	Palermo	Success in a few cases
Ballance	1900	London	Fistula in semicircular canal

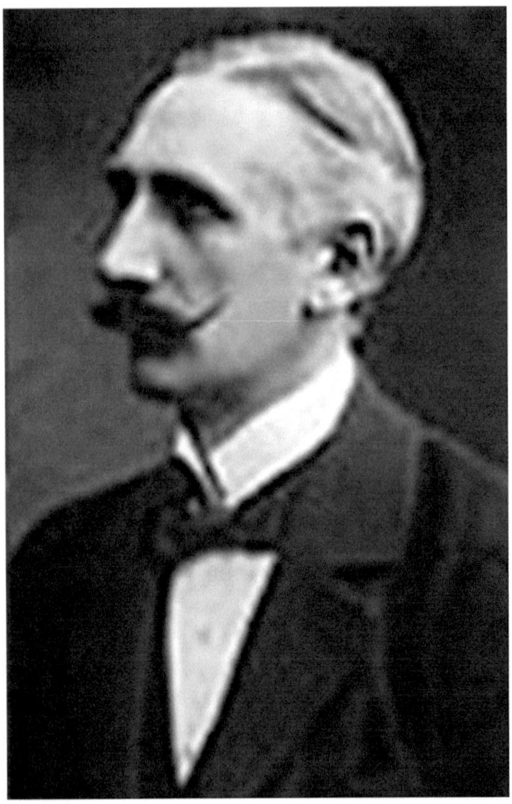

Fig. 1.6 Carl Pasow

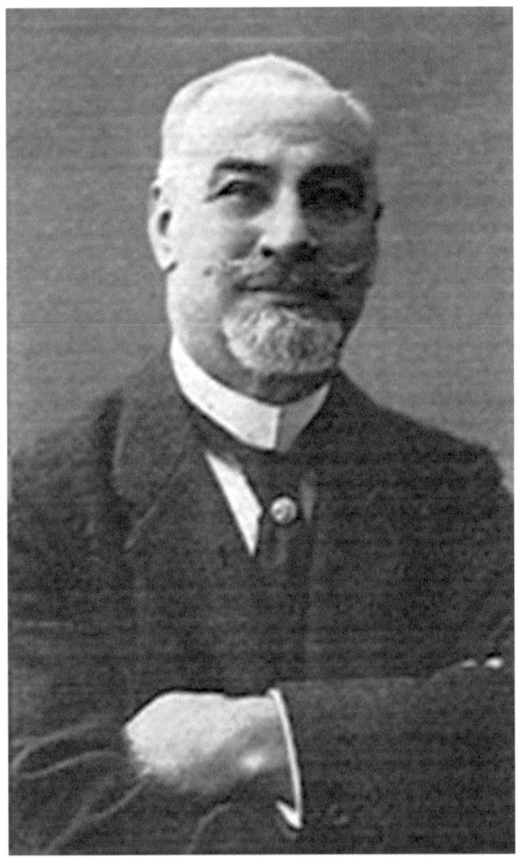

Fig. 1.7 Emile Moure

In 1894, on an international congress on medicine in Rome, V. Cozzolino (1853–1911), E. Moure (1855–1914) (Fig. 1.7), and A. Politzer condemned the surgery on the stapes in cases of otosclerosis. F. Bacon reports in his *Manual of Otology* (1898) that operations on the stapes should not be considered for a moment. In 1900, two other leading authorities at that time,

F. Siebenmann (1852–1928) and R.D. Botey (1855–1927), condemned the surgical treatment of otosclerosis at the International Congress of Otology again in Rome. In that pre-antibiotics era, an operation for hearing loss with the possible side effect of often fatal meningitis was the reason not to perform the surgery for hearing improvement in otosclerosis anymore. Politzer stated, also in 1900, that the simple mobilization of the stapes only results in a temporary effect on the hearing and that operative extraction of the stapes was of no use and could even be dangerous. In 1904, A. Denker (1863–1941) from Munich declared that there was no future for the surgical treatment of deafness due to otosclerosis. Since these statements at the beginning of the twentieth century and the poor results at that time, stapes surgery was abandoned for almost more than two decades as treatment for otosclerosis.

Reference

1. Tange RA. The history of otosclerosis treatment. Amsterdam: Kugler Publications; 2014.

2 The Putative Role of Measles Virus in the Pathogenesis of Otosclerosis

Tamás Karosi and István Sziklai

2.1 Introduction

Otosclerosis is a unique inflammatory bone remodeling disorder of the human otic capsule with a complex, but still partly unknown etiopathogenetic background [1–3]. Otosclerotic foci develop solely in the human otic capsule and in the stapes footplate [1, 4, 5]. Around 90 % of the lesions are located adjacent to the anterior pole of the oval window leading to the fixation of stapes footplate and conductive hearing loss (CHL) as a consequence of pathologic bone apposition [1]. Bone lesions may also involve the pericochlear region causing progressive sensorineural hearing loss (SNHL), tinnitus, vertigo, or dizziness [1]. In the Caucasian white population, the prevalence of manifest otosclerosis is about 0.3–0.4 % of the whole population, 5–9 % of those with hearing loss, and 18–22 % of those with conductive hearing loss [1, 2, 6]. There are several hypotheses explaining the development of SNHL in otosclerosis [7–10]. The biomechanical model emphasizes the role of morphologic changes in the modiolus, helicotrema, and also in the pericochlear bone layer that result in modulated elasticity of the spiral ligament [1, 11, 12]. This may result in disturbed reactions during the audiologic analysis of bone conduction. At this time, the autoimmune–inflammatory model is widely accepted, which emphasizes the potential role of measles virus (MV)-induced overexpression of pro-inflammatory cytokines (TNF-alpha, RANK, RANKL, etc.) in the pathogenesis of SNHL incidental to otosclerosis [10, 13–17].

As we have previously mentioned, otosclerosis is a unique organotropic disease of the human otic capsule [1]. It is a strictly localized remodeling disorder in a bone, which has the slowest or almost missing turnover in the human skeleton [1, 3, 5]. This biphasic bone remodeling disorder begins with an increased bone resorption and formation of new bone containing high amounts of organic materials that is called active otosclerosis, while it ends by a calcified and hypocellular bone production, called inactive otosclerosis (Fig. 2.1) [1]. The process results in absolutely different bone morphology than the structure of the healthy otic capsule (Fig. 2.1). Otosclerosis was first described by Antonio Maria Valsalva in 1740 as a bony obliteration of the oval window causing ankylosis of the stapes footplate [18]. Later, Adam Politzer used the term otosclerosis for the first time in 1894 [19]. His excellent and pioneering histopathologic drawings exhibit the histopathologic features of otosclerotic foci of different histopathologic activity [19, 20].

T. Karosi, MD, HSc, PhD (✉)
Department of Otolaryngology and Head and Neck Surgery, B-A-Z County Hospital and University Hospital, Szentpéteri Kapu 72-76, Miskolc 3526, Hungary
e-mail: karositamas@gmail.com

I. Sziklai
Department of Otolaryngology and Head and Neck Surgery, Clinical Center, University of Debrecen, Debrecen, Hungary

I. Sziklai (ed.), *Surgery of Stapes Fixations*, DOI 10.1007/978-3-319-28576-4_2

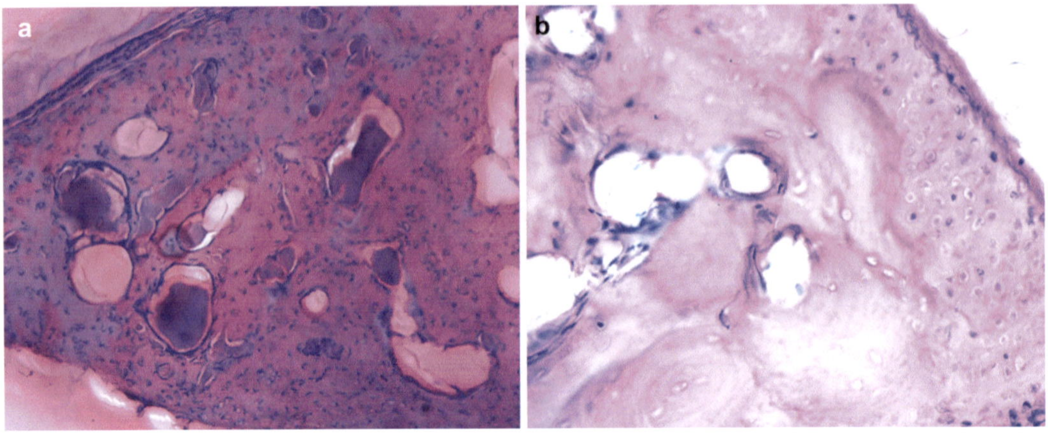

Fig. 2.1 Histopathology of stapedial otosclerotic foci (H.E.). (**a**) Active focus of otosclerosis at the anterior pole of the stapes footplate (40×). (**b**) Large magnification view of an inactive otosclerotic lesion involving the whole stapes footplate (100×)

2.1.1 Special Features of Otosclerosis

Otosclerosis shows several characteristic features. It occurs only in human [1–4]. This is why real animal model of this disease does not exist [1, 4]. Furthermore, it is not a generalized bone disease, since it develops only in the otic capsule and in the stapes footplate which have common embryonic origin [1]. Otosclerosis begins in the early adulthood, mostly in the third decades. The disease is usually bilateral and its incidence has a female dominancy (female/male ratio is 3.2) [1]. This suggests an autoimmune background of the disease since autoimmune diseases display significantly higher incidence among females [2, 21–30]. It should be noted that otosclerosis in childhood is not an existing clinical entity [1, 4]. Young patients (under 14 years of age) with stapes fixation usually suffer from other disease than otosclerosis, such as congenital stapes ankylosis, noggin mutation, and middle ear malformation, and mechanisms have been suggested as etiopathogenetic factors of the stapes fixation [1, 2, 21, 24, 28, 37–40]. Genetic background has long been suspected because inherited nature of this disorder was recognized already in the early twentieth century [1, 41, 42]. Inheritance, however, can only be found in the minority of the cases [1, 41, 42]. Sporadic occurrence is more frequently seen [1, 41, 42].

From the pathologic point of view, initial active phase of otosclerosis should be considered as the disease-specific phase. Inactive otosclerosis is only a consequence and "healing" of early active stages [31–33]. The inactive phase of the disease is a reparative process that fills up the pathologic pseudovascular cavities by newly formed and highly calcified bone [31–33, 43–45]. According to the current classification, active otosclerosis is represented by wide pseudovascular spaces filled with increased numbers of large, misshapen, and multinucleated osteoclasts. The osteoid contains small monomorphic cells that can be considered as osteoblasts (Fig. 2.1) [31–33]. Advanced, inactive stages of otosclerosis are featured by obliterated vascular and pseudovascular spaces and resorption lacunae with decreased numbers of osteoclasts and osteoblasts (Fig. 2.1) [31–33]. The normal hyaline cartilage layer of the stapes footplate toward the vestibule is destroyed by the otosclerotic lesion. Vanished chondrocytes in the peripheral zone are represented as empty cellular halos (Fig. 2.1) [31–33]. The activity of an individual otosclerotic focus does not show full correspondence with the clinical activity and symptoms of otosclerosis itself [1, 2, 31–33, 46]. Since otosclerosis is a multifocal disease, otic capsule might contain several foci of osteolysis with different histopathologic activities [1, 2, 31–33, 46].

2.1.2 Otosclerosis and Non-otosclerotic Stapes Fixations

Otosclerotic stapes ankylosis should be strictly distinguished from non-otosclerotic fixations [32–34, 36]. This can only be established by histopathologic examination of the stapes footplate specimens removed during stapes surgery (stapedectomy or partial stapedectomy) [32–34, 36]. Since most ear surgeons prefer stapedotomy to treat the conductive hearing loss due to otosclerosis; at this time it is quite difficult to obtain stapes footplate fragments containing the ankylosing lesion. Therefore, in most cases, ear surgeons have to rely with the diagnosis of otosclerosis (stapes ankylosis) on the patients' history, audiologic and CT (high resolution (HRCT) or cone beam (CBCT)) findings, and on the intraoperative observations [47, 48]. Since approximately one-third of stapes fixation cases turned out to belong to the group of non-otosclerotic fixations in our series of more than 1,300 consecutively removed stapes footplates by stapedectomy, it is important to stress that basic science research on the pathomechanism of otosclerosis can be performed only in histologically confirmed otosclerosis cases [31, 34, 36]. As compared to postoperative or postmortem histologic findings, HRCT or CBCT scanning of the temporal bone gives lower sensitivity and specificity of the diagnosis and can result in misinterpretation of the pathologically different stapes fixations [47, 48].

2.2 Remodeling in Normal and in Otosclerotic Bone

Normal bone remodeling in the petrous bone is characterized by a very slow osteolysis, which is in balance with the new bone formation. As to simplify this process, osteolysis is performed by mature osteoclasts, while osteosynthesis is the function of osteoblasts [1, 2]. Osteoclasts originate from bone marrow precursor cells and belong to the monocyte–macrophage system (MMS). These cells can be considered as real antigen-presenting cells (APC) [1]. On the other hand, osteoblasts can also derive from mesenchymal precursors, which also can differentiate into osteocytes [1, 2]. Physiologically, a sensitive equilibrium of osteolysis and new bone formation is controlled by a complex system, which involves endocrine, inflammatory, and local bone-specific regulatory processes [1, 2, 49]. Present time, the complex regulatory pathways of bone metabolism are reported as osteoimmunology [2]. The most important pathway in osteoimmunology is the TNF-alpha (tumor necrosis factor-alpha)–RANK (receptor activator of nuclear factor kappa B)–RANKL (RANK ligand)–OPG (osteoprotegerin) axis that preserves a fine regulation of osteointegrity by agonist and antagonist effects [50–52]. There are several other cytokines and paracrine mediators that might play an important role in the regulatory processes, such as TGF-beta (transforming growth factor-beta), BMP (bone morphogenetic protein), Wnt–beta catenin, etc. [53–58].

An imbalance or uncoupling of these two processes can be seen in otosclerosis [1, 2, 59–61]. Osteoclasts are multinucleated cells formed by the fusion of the progenitors of monocyte/macrophage family. Their principal function is bone resorption. In contrast, osteoblasts are bone-forming cells with equally important role in physiologic bone turnover [1, 2, 59–61]. The resorptive and bone-forming processes run simultaneously and maintain the physiologic balance of bone metabolism [1, 62–65]. Receptor activator of nuclear factor kappa B ligand (RANKL) is expressed and secreted by a variety of cells, including osteoblasts. RANKL facilitates the differentiation, activation, and survival of osteoclasts by the activation of its specific receptor RANK, which is located on osteoclasts [52, 53]. According to animal studies, osteopetrosis develops in RANKL-deficient mice showing absence of osteoclasts [44, 52, 53, 66]. Systemic application of RANKL in normal mice results in osteoporosis [44, 66].

Osteoprotegerin (OPG) is a powerful inhibitor of bone resorption and attenuates osteoclastogenesis [67–69]. OPG is a soluble decoy receptor that competes with RANK for RANKL. Due to the presence of RANK in osteoclasts and their precursors, OPG inhibits the differentiation, survival, and fusion of osteoclastic precursor cells and suppresses the activation of osteoclasts and promote their apoptosis [67–69]. In otosclerosis, high expression levels of OPG mRNA were detected in the spiral ligament, supporting cells of the organ of Corti and interdental cells of the spiral limbus [53, 67–70]. In contrast, no OPG expression could be detected within the bone of the otic capsule using immunohistochemistry [67–70]. Elevated concentrations of OPG were found in the perilymph [67–70]. Thus, OPG may be produced in the soft tissues of the cochlea and secreted into the perilymph and into the lacunar–canalicular system of the otic capsule. Diffusion of OPG from the perilymph into the surrounding bone is intensive. Probably, this is one of the reasons why the otic capsule is unique in its morphology and development [60].

In the human otic capsule, the bone turnover is under the total control of OPG, which shows extremely high concentration in the three layers (endosteal, middle embryonic, periosteal) of this bony structure [60, 67–70]. Therefore, bone remodeling is totally absent [1]. It is supposed that the source of OPG production is the stria vascularis that is an adjacent structure to the otic capsule [67–70]. Since the membranous labyrinth (cochlear duct, organ of Corti, and vestibular organs) is located within the otic capsule, its original structure should be preserved in order to prevent any biomechanical changes leading to serious consequences in the peripheral auditory processing [44, 60, 67–70]. This biomechanical hypothesis is the mostly accepted explanation for the almost missing metabolic activity of the human otic capsule [1, 2, 44, 60].

The otic capsule consists of the stapes footplate and the labyrinthine bone that develops from the mesenchymal cartilage precursors of the neural crest [1, 8, 11]. Its ossification process is purely enchondral that differs from other parts of temporal bone that represent desmal or vascular types of ossification [1, 8, 11]. In contrast, the stapes superstructure develops from the cartilage of the second branchial arch, from the Reichert's cartilage [1, 8, 11]. The incus and the malleus have different embryonic origin. These ossicles develop from the Meckel's cartilage, which is a special structure of the first branchial or mandibular arch [1]. This difference between the development of the stapes footplate and the superstructure may be responsible for the uninvolvement of the superstructure in the otosclerotic bone remodeling disorder. Sometimes the otosclerotic focus located in the footplate extends so progressively that near-footplate superstructure is also involved in the remodeling process. However, the primary lesion is never formed in the superstructure first [1, 2].

During endochondral ossification, vascularization of the cartilage is the first step. The chondrocytes and chondroblasts, which are grouped in chondrons, start to relocate into lines [1, 2, 8, 11]. The chondrocytes undergo well-ordered and controlled phases of cell proliferation, maturation, and apoptosis [1, 2, 8, 11, 61]. Proliferative chondrocytes synthesize type II collagen and form a columnar structure in the middle layer of the human otic capsule [28, 29, 72, 73]. They then stop proliferation and become prehypertrophic chondrocytes that differentiate into postmitotic hypertrophic cells [1]. Hypertrophic chondrocytes mineralize the surrounding extracellular matrix. In other bones, this differentiation process is followed by the apoptotic death of hypertrophic chondrocytes, capillary invasion, and finally replacement of the cartilaginous matrix by trabecular bone. Hypertrophic chondrocytes play a pivotal role in coordinating chondrogenesis and osteogenesis, as hypertrophic chondrocytes provide a scaffold for subsequent formation of trabecular bone [1]. In contrast, in the human otic capsule, hypertrophic chondrocytes form the inner endosteal and the outer periosteal layers; however, at the end of this process, they do not undergo apoptosis [1, 61]. The remnants of hypertrophic chondrocytes compose the globuli interossei, which are structures of resting chondroid elements showing several embryonic phenotypes (Fig. 2.2) [1, 61, 71].

The normal bone remodeling is disturbed in otosclerosis by a local intrinsic predisposition, and the disease is induced by extrinsic etiologic factors. At this point in time, we do think that otosclerosis is a disease of an inflammatory bone remodeling disorder of the human otic capsule that is initiated by defective measles virus infection in susceptible patients with unclarified genetic background [1, 5, 8, 42, 74–76]. Intrinsic, constitutional predisposition includes some localized morphological, genetic, and embryologic features. Presence of embryonic cartilage is a unique phenomenon in adults, which occurs exclusively in the otic capsule in the human skeleton: *fissula ante fenestram*, *fissula post fenestram*, and *globuli interossei*. This is known for decades [1, 11, 13]. A recent observation is that the vestibular surface of the stapes footplate is covered also by embryonic-type cartilage containing CD51/61 (OFA, osteoclast functional antigen) expressing chondrocytes (Fig. 2.2) [71]. CD51/61 expression is the sign of embryonic nature of these cells. Although embryonic cartilage can be found in the petrous bone of all human individuals, otosclerosis is very seldom among oriental people [1]. Also, the incidence among Caucasian race humans is only 0.4 %. On the other hand, silent otosclerotic foci are much more common: histologic otosclerosis without clinical symptoms has been reported as 8–11 % in large unselected autopsy series [1, 2, 6]. These facts stress the significance of a potential genetic predisposition in the development of otosclerosis [76].

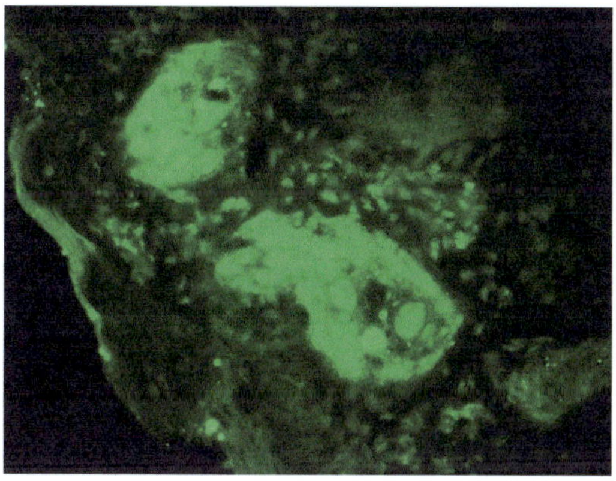

Fig. 2.2 CD51/61 (osteoclast functional antigen, OFA) expression in the central region of a histologically active otosclerotic focus located at the anterior pole of the stapes footplate (100×)

2.3 Measles Virus and Its General Receptor (CD46)

The etiologic role of measles virus arose in the past 25 years in the pathogenesis of otosclerosis [37–39]. Measles virus belongs to the paramyxovirus family [77]. It contains negative, single-stranded ribonucleic acid (ssRNA), which is replicated by the RNA polymerase enzymes of the infected cells (Fig. 2.3) [77]. Measles virus does not have neuraminidase (NA), but it contains fusion protein (FP), which plays an important role in syncytium formation (Fig. 2.3) [77].

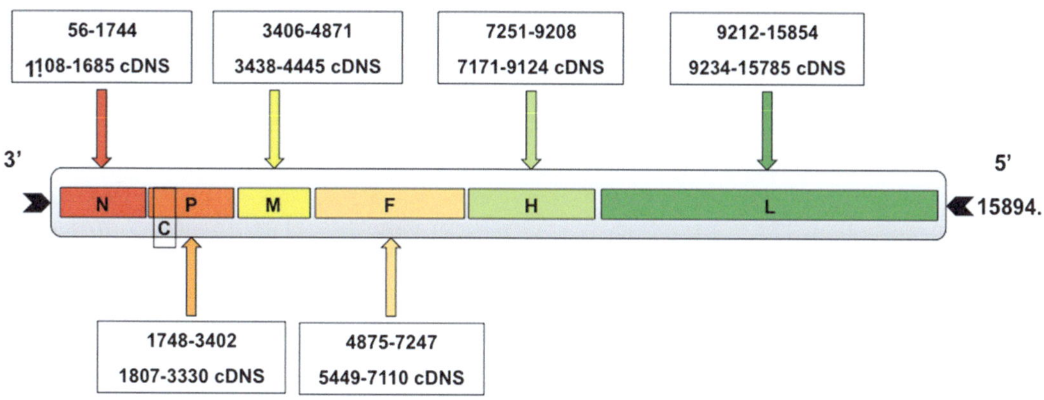

Fig. 2.3 The genomic structure of measles virus (negative single-stranded RNA, 3–5′). *N* nucleoprotein, *C* control protein, *P* phosphoprotein, *M* matrix protein, *H* hemagglutinin, *L* large protein

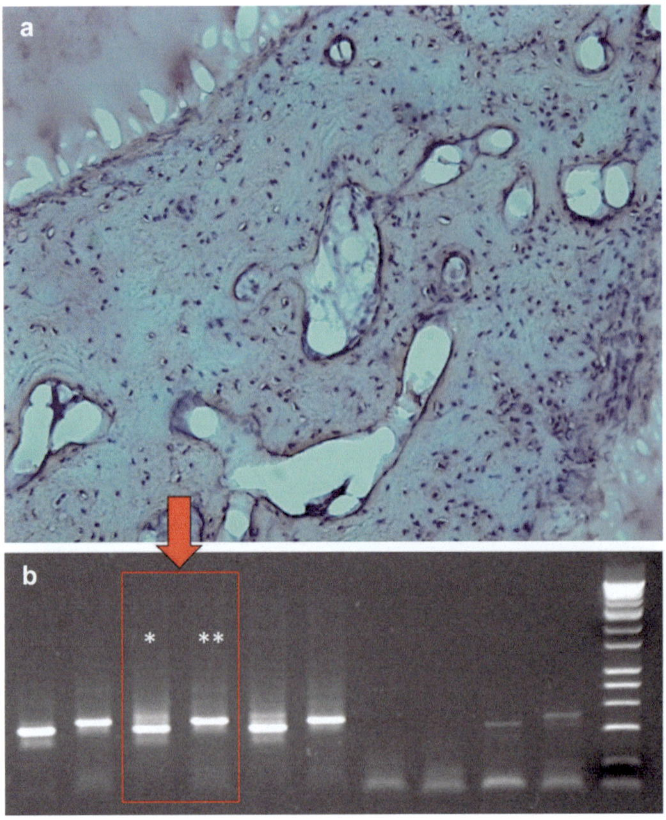

Fig. 2.4 Measles virus-specific RT-PCR in a histologically confirmed stapes footplate with active focus of otosclerosis. (**a**) Active otosclerotic lesion at the anterior pole of the stapes footplate (80×). (**b**) Nucleoprotein–RNA (NP)-specific RT-PCR revealed both positive reactions with different NP-specific primer pairs (221 bp, 231 bp)

Measles virus also has hemagglutinin (HG) and hemolysin (HL) (Fig. 2.3) [77]. The nucleoprotein (NP) and the matrix protein (MP) are necessary for the stabilization and for the replication of the viral RNA (Fig. 2.3) [77]. Measles virus is highly infective and has serious direct cytolytic effects that result in early necrosis of the infected cells [77]. However, in some cases, wild types (Edmonston, Schwartze, etc.) of measles virus may turn into defective infections causing special slow-virus-like diseases such as Paget's disease and subacute sclerosing panencephalitis (SSPE) [77]. Some researchers suppose otosclerosis as a slow-virus infection with a special genetic background of susceptibility [74, 75].

Arnold et al. have detected measles virus-specific immunoglobulin-G (IgG) in the perilymph samples obtained from patients with otosclerosis [78–82]. *McKenna* et al. recognized pleomorphic filamentous structures similar to paramyxovirus particles in the lesion-forming cells (osteoclasts, osteoblasts, endothelial cells) of otosclerotic foci by transmission electron microscopy (TEM) [38]. The presence of MP and NP of measles virus was also confirmed in the surgically removed stapes and postmortem cochlear samples of otosclerotic patients [81, 83–85]. A large amount of measles virus-derived proteins were detected on the surface of osteoclasts, fibroblasts, embryonic chondrocytes, and the proliferating endothelial cells (i.e., fusion protein, matrix protein, and hemagglutinin) by immunohistochemistry [81, 83–85]. Lower anti-measles IgG titers were measured in the serum samples of otosclerotic patients compared with control population [86, 87]. The presence of measles virus-derived RNA fragments in otosclerotic stapes footplates was also shown by RT-PCR (Fig. 2.4) [88–90]. However, there are some conflicting results. The RT-PCR method applied by Grayeli et al. revealed an absence of measles virus RNA in otosclerotic bone [91].

No animal model exists for the otosclerotic bone remodeling disorder, which is associated to the presence of measles virus in the foci [1, 87, 88]. Measles virus is found exclusively in otosclerotic bone in human [35, 87, 88]. This called the attention to the CD46 molecule, which is not expressed as measles virus receptor in any other mammalian species, except humans [92–96].

The general receptor of measles virus is the CD46, also known as membrane cofactor protein (MCP) [92–96]. CD46 has cofactor activity for inactivation of complement components C3b and C4b by serum factor I (SF-I), which protects the host cell from damage by the complement system [97–99]. Signals mediated by CD46 have great influence on T-cell activation [97–101]. CD46 plays a role in the pathogenesis of various inflammatory disorders. Its therapeutic potential in inflammatory diseases has also been suggested. Elevated serum levels of CD46 have been reported in systemic lupus erythematosus (SLE) [102]. High expression of CD46 has been detected in salivary glands of patients with Sjögren's syndrome [102]. Recombinant soluble CD46 has been introduced to animal models of various inflammatory diseases [102]. For example, CD46 treatment inhibited acute cardiac transplant rejection [103, 104]. Accordingly, targeted therapies using recombinant CD46 may be useful in autoimmune–inflammatory conditions [103, 104].

The mRNA of CD46 is translated from a single gene linked to chromosome 1q32; however, it is posttranslationally modified by alternative splicing resulting in 14 known splicing variants and corresponding protein isoforms [97–101]. Different numbers of CD46 isoforms are co-expressed by all nucleated human cells in various patterns [97–101]. However, specific functions have not been associated to isoform co-expression yet [92–96]. Exons 1–6 provide the conservative region, which determines the measles virus and HHV-6 receptor binding sites of CD46 [92–96]. Exons 7–9 encode the STP (serine–threonine–proline-rich) domain, which plays an important role in the anchoring to the extracellular matrix [92–96]. Exons 7–9 and 13 form the hypervariable region [92–96]. The transmembrane domain is encoded by exons 11–12 [92–96]. Common isoforms (*a-l*) of CD46 are associated with two frequent types of cytoplasmic domains: a shorter CYT-1 and a longer CYT-2 [92–96]. Isoforms *m* and *n* are featured by two rare cytoplasmic tails with unclear signaling process: CYT-3 and CYT-4 [92–96]. Type CYT-1 contains both casein kinase-2 and protein kinase-C phosphorylation sites, while CYT-2 has *src* kinase and casein kinase-2 phosphorylation sites indicating different signalization of CD46 isoforms having CYT-1 or CYT-2 cytoplasmic domains [92–96].

In the CD4-positive T lymphocytes, cross-linking of CD46 induces *vav* and *rac* activation and also the phosphorylation of *erk*-activated kinase, p120, and LAT adapter proteins [97–101]. This process results in T-cell receptor-dependent proliferation and induction of CD4-positive T cells [97–101]. Signals mediated by CD46 have greater effectiveness on T-cell activation than those mediated by CD3 and CD28 [97–101]. Measles virus binds to the CCP (complement control protein) region of CD46 [97–101]. Measles-activated CD46 associates to moesin that leads to the inhibition of interleukin-12 production [97–101]. This process induces the production of IL-12 p40, which regulates the proportion of T-helper 1 and 2 lymphocytes in the early stage of an immune response [97–101].

2.4 The Role of CD46 in the Pathogenesis of Otosclerosis

The average life span of an active otosclerotic focus is about 5–7 years until inactivation; hence, a dynamic genetic hypothesis is necessary to explain this "healing" process [1, 2, 75, 76]. The involvement of viral antigens, T cells, inflammatory cytokines, and other mediators in otosclerosis suggests an autoimmune–inflammatory nature of the disease [2, 75].

Specific diseases have not yet been attributed to CD46 isoform co-expression; however, previous studies supplied essential information about novel splicing variants of CD46 emphasizing a potential association between isoform co-expression and otosclerosis (Fig. 2.5) [75]. To our knowledge, our previous study was the first

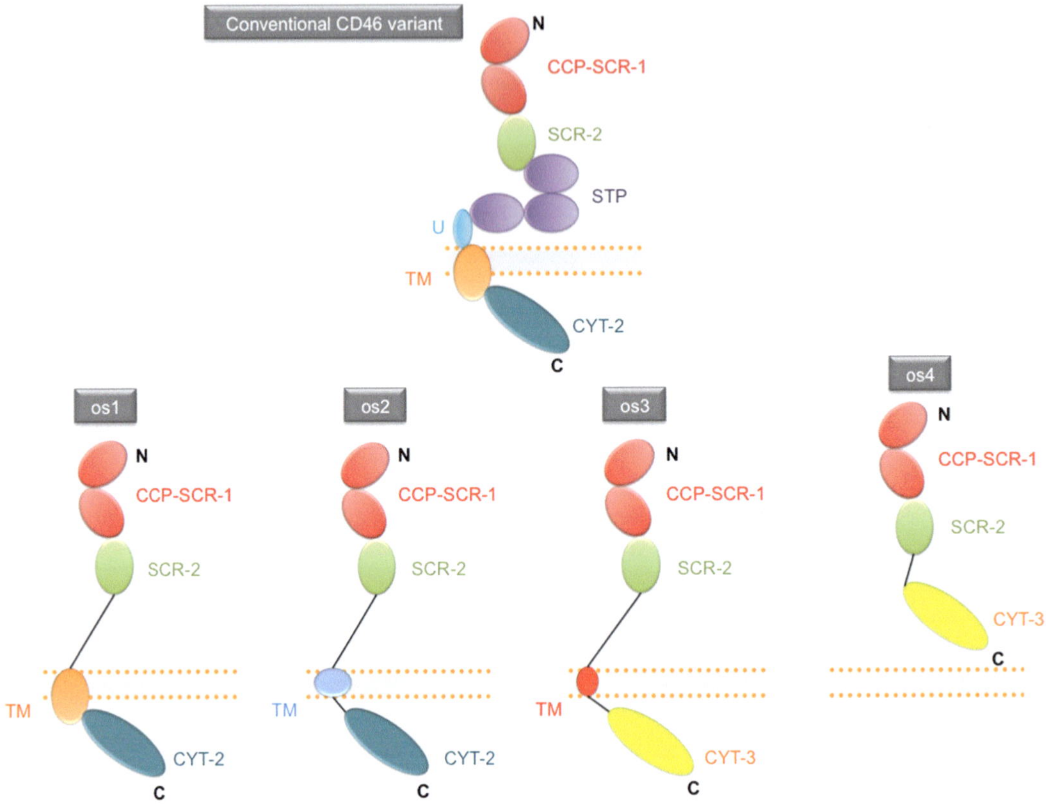

Fig. 2.5 Schematic model of otosclerosis-associated, new protein variants of CD46 molecule. *N* N terminal, *C* C terminal, *CCP* complement control protein, *SCR* short consensus repeats, *STP* serine–threonine–proline-rich region, *U* region of unknown significance, *TM* transmembrane region, *CYT* cytoplasmic domain

comprehensive report examining simultaneously the protein expression pattern of different CD46 variants in otosclerotic, non-otosclerotic, and normal stapes footplates to establish disease-associated alternative splicing (Figs. 2.5 and 2.6) [74, 75].

Various expressions of different splicing variants of CD46 seem to be the most acceptable explanation for the genetic background of otosclerosis [74, 75]. Newly described CD46 protein isoforms have shorter or missing transmembrane and uncommon cytoplasmic domains; however, virus-binding domain remains conservative (Fig. 2.5) [75]. Transmembrane and soluble isoforms of CD46 protein have been identified in humans and in transgenic mice [75]. In mice, there is an exon spliced alternatively, which allows to encode a soluble, cytoplasmic isoform [97–99]. Although soluble isoforms of human CD46 have been found in different body fluids, mRNA encoding soluble forms remains unidentified until now [75]. Previous studies supplied direct evidence of a human soluble CD46 isoform (*os4*) produced by alternative splicing (Fig. 2.5) [75]. These changes should result in functional consequences of signaling that may be responsible for the persisting replication of measles virus [75, 97–101].

Anti-measles IgG level is significantly decreased in the sera of patients with otosclerosis [86, 87]. Decreased production of anti-measles IgG is characteristic for otosclerosis, which is independent from vaccination or measles virus infection; and can be determined by expression of otosclerosis-associated CD46 isoforms [74, 75, 86, 87]. Newly described splicing variants of CD46 are supposed to allow virus internalization without TCR-dependent activation of primary

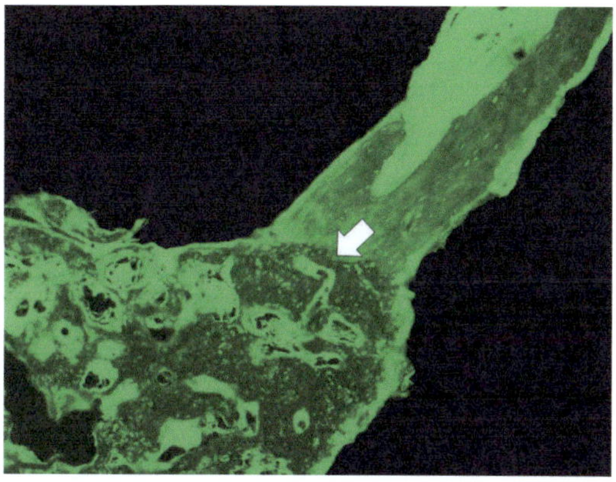

Fig. 2.6 CD46-specific immunofluorescent assay (IFA) in a stapes footplate with histologically active otosclerosis (60×). The *white arrow* displays the sharp border between the otosclerotic lesion and normal bone substance

CD4-positive T-helper cells and consecutive induction of B-cell-dependent immunoglobulin production [75, 97–101]. It is supposed that the most important factor in the pathogenesis of otosclerosis is a consecutive autoimmune reaction due to continuous CD46-presented viral antigen stimulation of natural killer cells and CD8-positive T lymphocytes [1, 2, 75]. Overexpression of TNF-alpha receptors (TNFRI/II) has been reported in active stages of otosclerosis, which highlights the inflammatory cascade due to activation of cellular immune system [1, 2]. Nevertheless, several inflammatory cytokines (TNF-alpha, IL-1, TGF-beta) and bone-specific proteins (osteoprotegerin, BMP, DDST) also may play a secondary promoting role in this process [1, 2].

Proteins expressed as different splicing isoforms are able to imitate regular Mendelian inheritance [75, 92–96]. Familial cases of otosclerosis showing obscure autosomal dominant inheritance with incomplete penetrance might be considered as a disease caused by unique alternative splicing of measles virus receptors in the otic capsule [75]. An unresolved question is whether measles virus can induce the expression of new CD46 splicing variants or existing novel isoforms lead to the increased virus affinity and smooth virus replication. We do think the answer is hidden in the expression of different regulatory proteins of alternative splicing leading to a special expression pattern and altered functions of CD46 that could explain the organ-specific and virus-associated pathogenesis of otosclerosis [1, 2, 75].

Active otosclerosis is featured by increased number of osteoclasts showing strong CD46 expression and high alkaline phosphatase activity (Fig. 2.6) [74]. In virus-negative, non-otosclerotic stapes fixations and in normal stapes footplates, a weak CD46 immunoreaction was demonstrated on the osteocytes and fibroblasts [74]. Nevertheless, chondrocytes of the stapediovestibular hyaline cartilage layer showed strong CD46-specific immunoreactions, respectively [74]. According to the previously mentioned considerations about the role of CD46, intense CD46-specific immunoreaction could relate to active virus replication, continuous receptor internalization, and chronic stimulation of the cellular immune system in otosclerosis [75, 97–101].

The humoral immune response of patients with otosclerosis seems permissive to a persistent viral replication, because anti-measles IgG level is significantly decreased in sera of these patients [86, 87]. This permissive feature may indicate an underlying genetic predisposition in otosclerosis [75, 76]. This can be related to the expression of otosclerosis-specific CD46 splicing variants, since their internalization may trigger signaling pathways leading to, e.g., silencing T lymphocytes and subsequently B lymphocytes [75, 97–101]. Cross-linking of CD46 isoforms downregulates IL-12 production, via unknown mechanisms [97–101]. Since, IL-12 plays an important role in immunoglobulin production and memory B-cell reactivation, this process may interfere with humoral immune response [86, 87, 97–101]. In contrast, *Avota* et al. have reported that ligation of CD46 is unlikely to contribute to measles virus-induced T-cell silencing, since wild-type strains do not interact with this molecule [105]. According to the current consensus, CD150 and CD46 may contribute in shaping T-cell responses, since they are able to change cytokine production [97–101].

As it was mentioned, otosclerosis-specific CD46 variants have short or missing transmembrane domains, which may imply faster virus internalization into the lesion-forming cells (Fig. 2.5). This may lead to a rapid antigen presentation and simultaneously to produce signaling molecules, which induce the silencing of cytotoxic T cells. This results in subsequent ligation of B lymphocytes, which is detected by the characteristic low anti-measles IgG serum level in otosclerotic patients [75, 86, 87]. The measles virus-binding cells and cytotoxic T lymphocytes serve with the underlying cellular background to the localized inflammatory process. Furthermore, otosclerosis-associated splicing variants of measles binding CD46 receptor are not expressed in the stapes of healthy individuals (Figs. 2.5 and 2.6) [74, 75]. A special expression pattern of CD46 isoforms due to organ-specific alternative splicing may explain genetically determined susceptibility for persisting measles virus infection observed in otosclerosis [78, 80].

2.5 Etiopathogenetic Models for Otosclerosis

Genetic predisposition for otosclerosis has long been disputed over the last decades, without obvious target genes or mutations to show up [1, 2, 76]. Several studies have reported genetic associations in populations with clinical otosclerosis – stapes fixation indeed – without histopathologic confirmation. These observations irrespected the possibility of non-otosclerotic fixations [76, 106–112]. The majority of genetic studies on families with stapes fixation and on large unselected populations have suggested an autosomal dominant mode of inheritance with incomplete penetrance of approximately 40–45 % [76, 109]. Genetic linkage studies have demonstrated the presence of eight loci [OTSC1, OTSC2, OTSC3, OTSC4, OTSC5, OTSC6, OTSC7, OTSC8] located on chromosomes 15q, 7q, 6p, 16q, 3q, 6q, and 9p, respectively [106–112]. Although these loci have been mapped, no causative genes and proteins have been identified, and we have little idea of the molecular process involved in this disease [42, 76, 106–112]. It has been reported that *COL1A1*, *BMP2*, *BMP4*, *TGFB1*, and *RELN* genes may also contribute to the development of otosclerosis [56–59, 113–117]. Furthermore, prior associations with these genes account for only a small fraction of the relative risk for otosclerosis or other types of stapes fixation [113–117]. These associations reported earlier cannot explain female dominancy, adult onset, organ specificity, and the inflammatory bone remodeling disorder as characteristic features of otosclerosis [1, 2].

Extrinsic factors may be infective, inflammatory, toxic, pharmacologic, and/or immunologic agents or mechanisms [1, 2]. Out of these, autoimmunity against embryonic cartilage type II collagen has already been considered [2, 27–30]. Others did not confirm this theory [1, 2, 12, 13]. Infection as a possible precipitating factor is addressed since *McKenna* discovered virus-like particles in the otosclerotic bone by transmission electron microscopy [38]. Others confirmed this and the virus was identified as measles [78–90]. N, H, and F proteins of the virus could be detected in the cytoplasm of the osteoblasts, chondroblasts, and macrophages by immunohistochemistry [78–90]. A virus-induced inflammatory process fits well to the histologic characteristics of otosclerotic bone in the active, osteolytic phase. It can be assumed that measles virus infection might persist in genetically susceptible individuals leading to a local inflammation. This is followed by a genetically determined bone remodeling disorder in the otic capsule (Fig. 2.7). Proteins or RNA of the measles virus cannot be demonstrated by anyone of the researchers in other bone samples than otosclerotic stapes footplate. Stapes footplates in non-otosclerotic stapes fixations do not contain measles RNA as well (Fig. 2.4) [78–90].

In otosclerosis, during the active phase, bone resorption lacunae develop in the vicinity of the measles-infected embryonic chondroblasts/chondrocytes. Embryonic chondrocytes were also demonstrated in the stapediovestibular interface where the footplate is covered by hyaline cartilage. Also, CD51/61 labeling could be demonstrated in chondrocytes of the annular ligament (Fig. 2.2) [71]. Embryonic chondrocytes in the footplate do express the measles virus-binding receptor, the CD46 (Fig. 2.6) [74, 75].

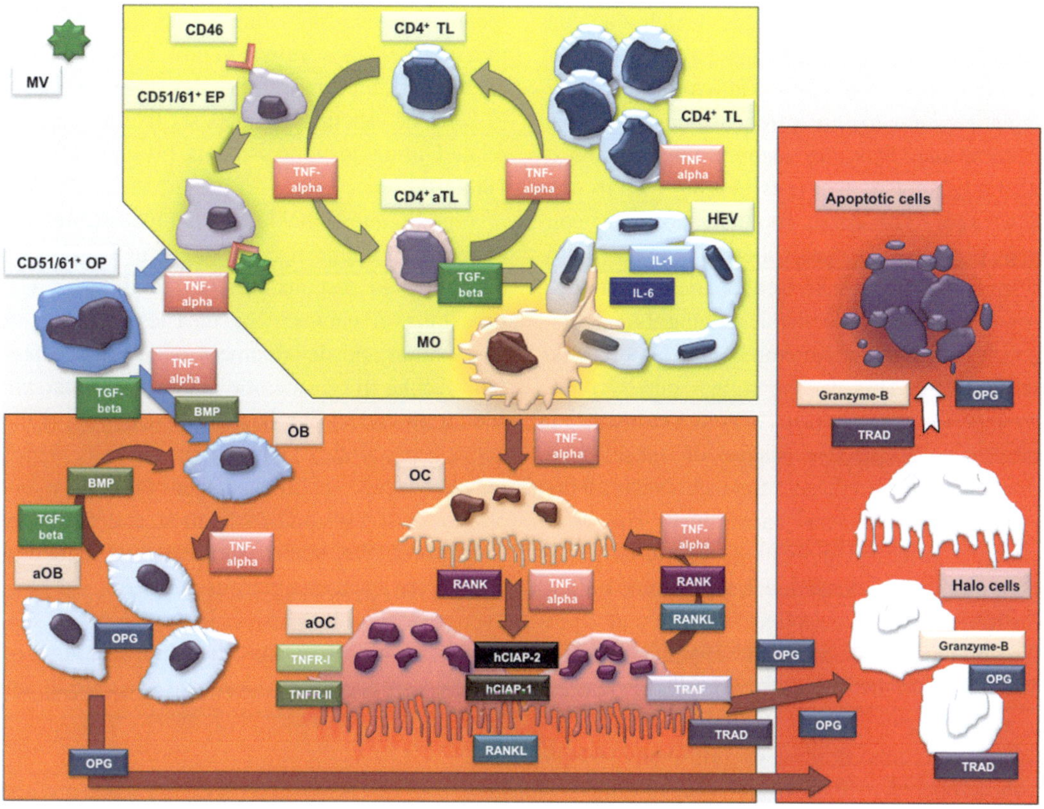

Fig. 2.7 Etiopathogenetic model for otosclerosis. *MV* measles virus, *MO* monocyte, *HEV* high endothelial venule, *TL* T lymphocyte, *EP* embryonic precursor, *OP* osteoid precursor, *OB* osteoblast, *OC* osteoclast, *aOB* activated osteoblast, *aOC* activated osteoclast

All nucleated cells contain this molecule in human. No other mammalian species express it. This can be the reason of the missing animal model for otosclerosis. The measles-infected chondrocytes in the stapes footplate recruit CD4+ and CD8+ cytotoxic T lymphocytes. The presence of CD4+ and CD8+ T lymphocytes in the otosclerotic foci were demonstrated [79, 81]. These T cells do not destroy the measles antigen-presenting chondrocytes for some presently unknown reasons. Rather, CD4+/CD8+ T cells produce TNF-alpha, a pro-inflammatory cytokine, which promotes maturation of osteoclasts from their precursor cells. Another putative way of forming otosclerotic lesion is that the measles-infected chondrocytes recruit not only CD4+/CD8+ T cells, but macrophages as well. Macrophages may serve as precursor cells for osteoclastic differentiation (Fig. 2.7).

However, a contradiction can be seen between reports about the presence of osteoclasts in the otosclerotic foci. Some researchers state that in active otosclerosis (otospongiosis), only few osteoclasts can be seen or there are no osteoclasts at all [79, 81]. *Arnold* denotes macrophages instead of osteoclasts indicating that macrophages may be the source of developing mature osteoclasts [79, 81]. The lesion-forming cell type should be clarified in the future. The otosclerotic foci contain multinucleated cells, which are embryonic in their phenotype (Fig. 2.2). These can be derived from chondroblasts, monocytes, or macrophages. Due to the very strong correlation between otosclerosis and measles virus presence, the lesion-forming cells should be derived from those cells as precursors, which are localized exclusively in the otic capsule and exhibit CD46 expression [74, 75]. This, however, does not exclude macrophages, which also contain CD46 receptors. Still it is interesting to know how long is it necessary for macrophages to differentiate into mature osteoclast in the human otic capsule. This may respond the question of why otosclerosis manifests hearing loss in only adult ages. The stapes footplate normally contains Haversian lacunae, whereas in inactive otosclerosis, the resorption lacunae are filled up by a newly formed, hypocellular, and highly calcified bone. This bone is structured in a lamellar-like morphology. This can be shown out by phase contrast microscopy (Fig. 2.1). It means that in histologically inactive stages of otosclerosis, osteoclasts, macrophages, and osteoblasts all disappear from the osteoid background. This "vanishing" process might be coordinated by programmed cell death due to the chronic inflammation and uncontrolled release of pro-inflammatory cytokines (TNF-alpha, RANK, RANKL, TGF-beta) [54, 55, 60, 61].

A significant decrease in the incidence of otosclerosis is found in measles-vaccinated population compared to the gender- and age-matched unvaccinated population [82, 86, 87]. It is interesting to note, however, that otosclerosis develops in only those individuals, who do not respond to vaccination and hence do not produce anti-measles IgG [82, 86, 87]. Vaccination against measles or passing through a measles infection may cause a localized virus particle presence if specific binding receptors (CD46) exist. It is well known that vaccination against measles provides a milder seropositivity (serum anti-measles IgG level) than natural infection [82, 86, 87]. In populations of different countries, as high as >20 % of the vaccinated population exhibited negligible anti-measles IgG serum levels, which may indicate the necessity of a revaccination [82]. The low response rate to vaccination makes possible subclinical measles infection that can be the cause of a persistent measles virus presence in the affected individuals. Taking the approximately 0.4 % incidence of otosclerosis in the Caucasian population, an intrinsic predisposition, a probably genetic basis, should be responsible for the development of the disease in some individuals, whereas others will resist against the localized bone remodeling disturbance. The fact that otosclerosis develops in only those individuals who exhibit low anti-measles IgG serum level in spite of vaccination suggests that a measles-related immunosuppression is present [86, 87, 100, 101].

It is still questionable whether measles-related abnormal immune response or genetic immune deficiency is responsible for the disease. The time interval between the measles infection or vaccination and development of the first osteolytic lacuna in otosclerotic patients is unknown. Moderate conductive hearing loss is due to the active (spongiotic) phase of the disease, which may not exceed the 20–30 dB air-bone gap. When otosclerosis turns to inactivation and the bony fixation of the stapes footplate subsequently obtains the level of a serious ankylosis, the conductive hearing loss arrives to the 40–50 dB air-bone gap. It seems from the clinical course of otosclerosis that the development of a >30 dB air-bone gap takes decades [1, 2, 10, 47, 61].

2.6 Otosclerosis: A Measles Virus-Induced Osteoimmunologic Disease?

The normal otic capsule exerts very low levels of bone turnover and does not contain functioning osteoclasts [1, 2, 11, 13, 31, 32]. The histologic activity of otosclerotic foci may be categorized from active to completely inactive stages depending on the cellularity, degree of vascularization, amount of extracellular collagen matrix, and the presence of osteoblasts and osteoclasts (Fig. 2.1) [11, 13, 31, 32]. There are numerous osteoclasts, osteoblasts, fibroblasts, and endothelial cells in active otosclerotic lesions which can be responsible for the development of spongiotic structure. In response to this enhanced bone resorption, a regenerative process occurs in the foci causing fibrous transformation by osteoblasts (Fig. 2.1) [11, 13, 31, 32]. The early stages of otosclerosis have been associated with persisting measles virus infection and a consecutive inflammatory reaction. In brief, the active phase is characterized by incremental inflammation, detectable measles virus genome, and locally increased expression of TNF-alpha and OPG negativity. The inactive phase is featured by measles virus and OPG positivity, TNF-alpha negativity, and lack of signs of inflammation [16, 17].

Measles virus antigens are expressed on the surface of infected cells by the MHC-I molecules. Therefore, CD8+ T-cell-dependent immune responses lead to TNF-alpha release and subsequent bone resorption [9, 10, 16, 17]. This is the most viable theory, but activated monocytes, macrophages, B cells, T cells, and osteoclasts are also able to secrete TNF-alpha into the osteolytic foci, and thus they may further perpetuate the inflammatory events [10, 16, 17]. TNF-alpha is a pro-inflammatory cytokine that plays an essential role in the differentiation of bone marrow-derived mononuclear cells to osteoclasts and stromal cells to osteoblasts. This cytokine is also an indispensable paracrine mediator during intercellular communication between osteoclasts and osteoblasts. High levels of TNF-alpha stimulate osteoclast activation, induce RANKL expression, and decrease osteoclast apoptosis leading to osteolysis and spongiosis [8, 50–53]. TNF-alpha overproduction in otosclerosis further stimulates osteoclast formation through the dual action of inhibiting secretion of OPG and stimulating that of RANKL [50–53]. TNF-alpha may enter into the perilymph and cortilymph utilizing the same channels as OPG when migrating from the perilymph to the otic capsule. TNF-alpha may interfere with the electromotility of outer hair cells, leading to SNHL as a consequence of cochlear or far advanced otosclerosis [9, 10].

Increased expression of TNF-alpha receptors has been reported in otosclerosis [16, 17, 60, 61]. The type I TNF receptor (TNFRI) is universally expressed by all nucleated human cells, and its activation results in signal transduction via at least three different pathways [50–53]. The most important way of activation is mediated through nuclear factor kappa B (NF-kB), which directly leads to inflammatory cytokine production, inflammatory cell proliferation, and survival [50–53]. The second way is the complex activation cascade of the mitogen-activated protein kinase (MAPK) system, inducing intense cell multiplication and survival of cells [50–53]. The third way is the TNFRI-associated signalization leading to death domain-mediated and caspase-associated induction of apoptosis by the accumulation of cysteine protein caspase 8 complexes [50–53]. After reaching the critical concentration of caspase 8, apoptotic cell death occurs [50–53]. Type II TNF-alpha receptor (TNFRII) is expressed by lymphocytes, antigen-presenting cells, and osteoclasts. The activation of TNFRII plays an important role in the recruitment of immune cells, activation of osteoclasts, and production of inflammatory cytokines [50–53]. In active otosclerosis, early bone resorption is followed by increased bone formation and sclerosis. Recently, the wingless protein (Wnt)–b-catenin system has been implicated in osteoblast activation and new bone formation [118–124]. Sclerostin and the Dickkopf-1 (DKK-1) protein are inhibitors of Wnt and thus the bone formation [118–124]. Hence, apart from the RANKL/OPG system, the Wnt/DKK-1 sclerostin balance has also been implicated in bone remodeling. Interestingly, TNF-alpha does not only stimulate bone loss by inducing RANKL. It also induces DKK-1 and indirectly inhibits Wnt-mediated bone formation [118–124]. Although there is few information available on the role of Wnt–b-catenin/sclerostin–DKK-1 system in otosclerosis, Wnt and its target genes have been identified in the cochlea and in various other parts of the inner and middle ear [118–124]. High expression of Wnt and b-catenin have been associated with the development of the human otic capsule [118–124]. Finally, a mutation in the sclerostin (SOST) gene has been described leading to bone dysplasias, sclerosteosis, and conductive hearing loss due to "too much bone" in the middle ear [118–124].

It has been suggested that one of the most important factors in the pathogenesis of otosclerosis is a consecutive autoimmune reaction due to the continuous viral antigen stimulation of the cellular immune system [1, 2, 37]. Overexpression of TNF-alpha receptors in active stages of otosclerosis might induce an inflammatory osteolytic cascade [61]. Several inflammatory cytokines (TNF-alpha, IL-1, TGF-beta) and bone-specific proteins (OPG, BMP) may play a promoting role in this process [1, 2]. An increased expression of hCIAP1 and hCIAP2 apoptosis inhibitor proteins has been reported in otosclerosis [61]. This might be the molecular response to intense TNF-alpha release mediated by NK cells and osteoclasts in early stages of otosclerosis. TNF-alpha acts through its decoy receptors, activates the TNF-alpha receptor-associated factors (TRAF1 and TRAF2), and induces apoptosis due to activation of variable death domains. Inhibitors of apoptosis do not interact with TNF-alpha or TNF-alpha receptors but associate with TRAF1 and TRAF2 [61]. HCIAP1 and hCIAP2 can directly bind to TNF receptor-activated caspase-3 and caspase-7 and inhibit their proteolytic activities [50–53]. Overexpression of apoptosis inhibitors results in increased cell survival, proliferation, and extended osteoclast activation (Fig. 2.7). As to our previous results, the average life span of an active otosclerotic focus is about 5–7 years [10, 61]. During this period, TNF-alpha and the consecutive hCIAP response run down and result in decreased vascularization and moderate activity of osteoclasts (Fig. 2.7). The volume of osteoid substance increases, and osteolytic lacunae and pseudovascular spaces are eventually obliterated. Activated NK cells and CD8+ cytotoxic T lymphocytes show further accumulation in the perivascular spaces in the otosclerotic focus with decreasing activity. This stage is the "histological healing" of otosclerosis; however, on the molecular level, a severe cellular destruction can be considered due to granzyme b and perforin release from immune cells (Fig. 2.7) [61]. The molecular cascade of immune-mediated apoptosis starts, while increasing OPG production leads to further calcification [60, 61]. The woven and concentric structure of cement lines turns into lamellar pattern with marked thickening. The endpoint of the increased bone turnover is an apoptotic cell death with calcification and avascularization of the osteoid substance: burn out otosclerosis (Fig. 2.7) [31–33].

An important cytokine, TGF-beta, can be involved in the pathogenesis of otosclerosis [2, 8, 13, 54, 55]. TGF-beta is the most important growth factor in the human bone. It plays a critical role in inducing mesenchymal cell differentiation to osteoblasts. TGF-beta regulates osteoblast differentiation, matrix formation, tissue fibrosis, and mineralization. TGF-beta interacts with several molecular pathways in osteoblasts biology, such as the Wnt–b-catenin pathway [8, 13, 54, 55, 118–124]. As discussed above, otosclerosis is associated with fibrosis and new bone formation as repair mechanism following bone resorption [8, 13, 54, 55]. Bone morphogenetic proteins (BMPs) that also belong to the TGF-beta gene family have recently been implicated in the pathogenesis of otosclerosis [56–59].

It has been suggested that different types of BMP and their receptors may be involved in the pathologically increased bone turnover in otosclerosis [56–59]. *Lehnerdt* et al. have performed immunohistochemical analysis of BMPs and BMP receptors in otosclerotic stapes footplates [57, 58]. Significantly increased BMP2, BMP4, and BMP7 expression was demonstrated within the otosclerotic foci compared to normal and non-otosclerotic bone specimens [59]. Among BMP receptors, BMPR-1B and BMPR-2 showed increased immunoreactivity, whereas BMPR-1A always exerted negative reaction [57, 58]. Thus, the effects of BMPs may be mediated through type-1B and type-2 BMP receptors in otosclerosis [57, 58]. Later, the same group carried out immunofluorescent typing of different BMP isoforms in active otosclerotic tissues. Again, consequent expressions of BMP2, BMP4, and BMP7 were demonstrated [57–59]. *Schrauwen* et al. have reported the potential role of various BMP isoforms in the risk of otosclerosis [56]. There was a significant association between clinical otosclerosis and the increased expression of BMP2 and BMP4 [56]. The same authors reported two otosclerosis-associated single-nucleotide polymorphisms (SNPs) in the genes of BMP2 and BMP4 [56]. The first noncoding SNP rs3178250 (BMP2) was located into a 3′ untranslated region, while the second named as rs17563 (BMP4) led to amino acid exchange in BMP4 that was strongly associated to otosclerosis [56]. These observations are reasonable to assume, since both BMPs and TGF-beta are key regulators of new bone formation. In addition, there are several interconnected events in the BMP and TGF-beta pathways that result in inverse interactions between the two protein groups [55–59].

At this point, we have to return to the embryology of the otic capsule. As we have previously described, a regular enchondral ossification develops in the otic capsule and in the stapes footplate, which is completed after 1 year [1, 2]. Osteoblastic and osteoclastic activity, normally associated with bone turnover, is rarely, if ever, seen in the adult otic capsule [1]. The enchondral layer of the otic capsule contains peculiar, embryonic chondrocytes, which persist throughout life [1]. Similar cells can be found in the vestibular layer of the stapes footplate. It has been reported that these remnants may be the sites of the earliest otosclerotic foci [1, 2, 11–13]. However, these cells disappear from otosclerotic foci and replaced by pre-osteoclasts, active osteoclasts, and osteoblasts [11–13]. In contrast to normal adult otic capsule, osteoclasts and osteoblasts of otosclerotic foci express a special embryonic glycoprotein: CD51/61 [71]. In addition, increased expression of BMPs, TGF-beta, TNF-alpha, and apoptosis inhibitors (hCIAP1/2) also supports the embryonic chondrocyte reactivation hypothesis in otosclerosis [55–59, 61]. According to previous reports, chondroblasts and osteoblasts might be reactivated and transformed into osteoclasts due to the inflammatory response induced by measles virus infection [1, 2, 37].

Conclusions

Histologically proven otosclerotic stapes footplates removed during stapedectomy contain measles virus RNA fragments, without exception. As controls, non-otosclerotic and fixed (calcification, fibrosis, etc.) footplates do not contain virus RNA, without exception. The disease-specific first phase of otosclerosis (called active otosclerosis) can be histologically characterized as a spongiotic bone with resorption lacunae, which contain large multinucleated and small monomorphic cells. These lesion-forming cells are probably osteoclasts and osteoblasts. These cells exhibit high CD51/61-specific immunoreaction as sign of their embryonic nature. These cells also show very high immunofluorescence activity against CD46 antigen. This molecule is a specific measles virus-binding receptor, which is expressed very little in adult bone cells, and it is not expressed in any other mammalian species. Embryonic phenotype is also proven in chondrocytes of the annular ligament and the stapediovestibular surface of the healthy and non-otosclerotically fixed stapes footplates. These chondrocytes express CD46 measles receptor as well. The otosclerotic lesion-forming cells consequently may derive from embryonic chondrocytes. Otosclerotic bone contains disease-specific splicing isoforms of CD46, which were described exclusively in otosclerosis. Otosclerotic patients are anti-measles IgG-seronegative individuals after vaccination against measles. Seronegativity is found in >20 % of vaccinated people. The incidence of otosclerosis is, however, only 0.4 % in the Caucasian population. Prone to otosclerosis, consequently, is an unknown genetic predisposition for measles-related localized inflammatory bone resorption in the human otic capsule.

Declarations Authors have no conflicts of interest.

References

1. Chole RA, McKenna M. Pathophysiology of otosclerosis. Otol Neurotol. 2001;22:249–57.
2. Karosi T, Szekanecz Z, Sziklai I. Otosclerosis: an autoimmune disease? Autoimmun Rev. 2009;9:95–101.
3. Yoo TJ. Etiopathogenesis of otosclerosis: a hypothesis. Ann Otol Rhinol Laryngol. 1984;93:28–33.
4. McKenna MJ, Kristiansen AG. Molecular biology of otosclerosis. Adv Otorhinolaryngol. 2007;65:68–74.
5. Wang PC, Merchant SN, McKenna MJ, Glynn RJ, Nadol Jr JB. Does otosclerosis occur only in the temporal bone? Am J Otol. 1999;20:162–5.
6. Declau F, Van Spaendonck M, Timmermans JP, Michaels L, Liang J, Qiu JP, Van de Heyning P. Prevalence of otosclerosis in an unselected series of temporal bones. Otol Neurotol. 2001;22:596–602.

7. Gros A, Vatovec J, Sereg-Bahar M. Histologic changes on stapedial footplate in otosclerosis. Correlations between histologic activity and clinical findings. Otol Neurotol. 2003;24:43–7.
8. Stankovic KM, McKenna MJ. Current research in otosclerosis. Curr Opin Otolaryngol Head Neck Surg. 2006;14:347–51.
9. Sziklai I. Human otosclerotic bone-derived peptide decreases the gain of the electromotility in isolated outer hair cells. Hear Res. 1996;95:100–7.
10. Sziklai I, Batta TJ, Karosi T. Otosclerosis: an organ-specific inflammatory disease with sensorineural hearing loss. Eur Arch Otorhinolaryngol. 2009;266:1711–8.
11. Michaels L. The temporal bone: an organ in search of a histopathology. Histopathology. 1991;18:391–4.
12. Niedermeyer HP, Arnold W. Etiopathogenesis of otosclerosis. ORL J Otorhinolaryngol Relat Spec. 2002;64:114–9.
13. Cureoglu S, Schachern PA, Ferlito A, Rinaldo A, Tsuprun V, Paparella MM. Otosclerosis: etiopathogenesis and histopathology. Am J Otolaryngol. 2006;27:334–40.
14. Arnold W, Niedermeyer HP, Lehn N, Neubert W, Höfler H. Measles virus in otosclerosis and the specific immune response of the inner ear. Acta Otolaryngol. 1996;116:705–9.
15. Niedermeyer HP, Arnold W. Otosclerosis: a measles virus associated inflammatory disease. Acta Otolaryngol. 1995;115:300–3.
16. Karosi T, Jókay I, Kónya J, Szabó LZ, Pytel J, Jóri J, Szalmás A, Sziklai I. Detection of osteoprotegerin and TNF-alpha mRNA in ankylotic Stapes footplates in connection with measles virus positivity. Laryngoscope. 2006;116:1427–33.
17. Karosi T, Kónya J, Szabó LZ, Pytel J, Jóri J, Szalmás A, Sziklai I. Codetection of measles virus and tumor necrosis factor-alpha mRNA in otosclerotic stapes footplates. Laryngoscope. 2005;115:1291–7.
18. Valsalva A. De aurae humana tractatus. Venetiis. Joanne Baptista Margagnus. 1740.
19. Politzer A. Über primare erkrankung der knöchernen labyrinthkapsel. Z Ohrenheilk. 1894;25:309–27.
20. Guild SR. Histologic otosclerosis. Ann Otol. 1947;24:246–66.
21. Dahlqvist A, Diamant H, Dahlqvist SR, Cedergren B. HLA antigens in patients with otosclerosis. Acta Otolaryngol. 1985;100:33–5.
22. Miyazawa T, Tago C, Ueda H, Niwa H, Yanagita N. HLA associations in otosclerosis in Japanese patients. Eur Arch Otorhinolaryngol. 1996;253:501–3.
23. Bernstein JM, Shanahan TC, Schaffer FM. Further observations on the role of the MHC genes and certain hearing disorders. Acta Otolaryngol. 1996;116:666–71.
24. Sølvsten Sørensen M, Nielsen LP, Bretlau P, Jørgensen MB. The role of type II collagen autoimmunity in otosclerosis revisited. Acta Otolaryngol. 1988;105:242–7.
25. Joliat T, Seyer J, Bernstein J, Krug M, Ye XJ, Cho JS, Fujiyoshi T, Yoo TJ. Antibodies against a 30 kilodalton cochlear protein and type II and IX collagens in the serum of patients with inner ear diseases. Ann Otol Rhinol Laryngol. 1992;101:1000–6.
26. Bujía J, Alsalameh S, Jerez R, Sittinger M, Wilmes E, Burmester G. Antibodies to the minor cartilage collagen type IX in otosclerosis. Am J Otol. 1994;15:222–4.
27. Helfgott SM, Mosciscki RA, San Martin J, Lorenzo C, Kieval R, McKenna M, Nadol J, Trentham DE. Correlation between antibodies to type II collagen and treatment outcome in bilateral progressive sensorineural hearing loss. Lancet. 1991;337:387–9.
28. Yoo TJ, Shea Jr JJ, Floyd RA. Enchondral cartilage rests collagen-induced autoimmunity: a possible pathogenetic mechanism of otosclerosis. Am J Otolaryngol. 1987;8:317–24.
29. Harris JP, Woolf NK, Ryan AF. A reexamination of experimental type II collagen autoimmunity: middle and inner ear morphology and function. Ann Otol Rhinol Laryngol. 1986;95:176–80.
30. Jesić S, Radulović R, Arsović N. Altered immunoregulations in otosclerosis: presence of autoantibodies in otosclerotic sera samples. Eur Arch Otorhinolaryngol. 1997;254 Suppl 1:S50–2.
31. Iyer PV, Gristwood RE. Histopathology of the stapes in otosclerosis. Pathology. 1984;16:30–8.
32. Linthicum Jr FH. Histopathology of otosclerosis. Otolaryngol Clin N Am. 1993;26:335–52.
33. Schuknecht HF, Barber W. Histologic variants in otosclerosis. Laryngoscope. 1985;95:1307–17.
34. Karosi T, Kónya J, Petkó M, Szabó LZ, Pytel J, Jóri J, Sziklai I. Two subgroups of stapes fixation: otosclerosis and pseudo-otosclerosis. Laryngoscope. 2005;115:1968–73.
35. Karosi T, Kónya J, Petkó M, Sziklai I. Histologic otosclerosis is associated with the presence of measles virus in the stapes footplate. Otol Neurotol. 2005;26:1128–33.
36. Karosi T, Csomor P, Petkó M, Liktor B, Szabó LZ, Pytel J, Jóri J, Sziklai I. Histopathology of nonotosclerotic stapes fixations. Otol Neurotol. 2009;30:1058–66.
37. Arnold W, Friedmann I. Otosclerosis – an inflammatory disease of the otic capsule of viral aetiology? J Laryngol Otol. 1988;102:865–71.
38. McKenna MJ, Mills BG. Ultrastructural and immunohistochemical evidence of measles virus in active otosclerosis. Acta Otolaryngol Suppl. 1990;470:130–40.
39. Niedermeyer HP, Arnold W, Schuster M, Baumann C, Kramer J, Neubert WJ, Sedlmeier R. Persistent measles virus infection and otosclerosis. Ann Otol Rhinol Laryngol. 2001;110:897–903.
40. Horner KC. The effect of sex hormones on bone metabolism of the otic capsule – an overview. Hear Res. 2009;252:56–60.

41. Clayton AE, Mikulec AA, Mikulec KH, Merchant SN, McKenna MJ. Association between osteoporosis and otosclerosis in women. J Laryngol Otol. 2004;118:617–21.
42. Ealy M, Chen W, Ryu GY, Yoon JG, Welling DB, Hansen M, Madan A, Smith RJ. Gene expression analysis of human otosclerotic stapedial footplates. Hear Res. 2008;240:80–6.
43. Chevance LG, Bretlau P, Jorgensen MB, Causse J. Otosclerosis. An electron microscopic and cytochemical study. Acta Otolaryngol (Stockh) Suppl. 1970;272:1–44.
44. Zehnder AF, Kristiansen AG, Adams JC, Kujawa SG, Merchant SN, McKenna MJ. Osteoprotegrin knockout mice demonstrate abnormal remodeling of the otic capsule and progressive hearing loss. Laryngoscope. 2006;116:201–6.
45. Arnold W. Some remarks on the histopathology of otosclerosis. Adv Otorhinolaryngol. 2007;65:25–30.
46. Moscicki RA, San Martin JE, Quintero CH, Rauch SD, Nadol JB, Bloch KJ. Serum antibody to inner ear proteins in patients with progressive hearing loss. Correlation with disease activity and response to corticosteroid treatment. JAMA. 1994;272: 611–6.
47. Karosi T, Csomor P, Sziklai I. The value of HRCT in stapes fixations corresponding to hearing thresholds and histologic findings. Otol Neurotol. 2012;33:1300–7.
48. Marx M, Lagleyre S, Escudé B, Demeslay J, Elhadi T, Deguine O, Fraysse B. Correlations between CT scan findings and hearing thresholds in otosclerosis. Acta Otolaryngol. 2011,131.351–7.
49. Brookler K. Basis for understanding otic capsule bony dyscrasias. Laryngoscope. 2006;116:160–1.
50. Mannel DN, Echtenacher B. TNF in the inflammatory response. Chem Immunol. 2000;74:141–61.
51. Locksley RM, Killeen N, Lenardo MJ. The TNF and TNF receptor superfamilies: integrating mammalian biology. Cell. 2001;104:487–501.
52. Wajant H, Pfizenmaier K, Scheurich P. Tumor necrosis factor signaling. Cell Death Differ. 2003;10(1): 45–65.
53. Theoleyre S, Wittrant Y, Tat SK, Fortun Y, Redini F, Heymann D. The molecular triad OPG/RANK/RANKL: involvement in the orchestration of pathophysiological bone remodelling. Cytokine Growth Factor Rev. 2004;15(6):457–75.
54. Thys M, Schrauwen I, Vanderstraeten K, Dieltjens N, Fransen E, Ealy M, Cremers CW, van de Heyning P, Vincent R, Offeciers E, Smith RH, van Camp G. Detection of rare nonsynonymous variants in TGFB1 in otosclerosis patients. Ann Hum Genet. 2009;73:171–5.
55. Bodo M, Venti G, Baroni T, Bellucci C, Giammarioli M, Donti E, Paludetti G, Stabellini G, Carinci P. Phenotype of in vitro human otosclerotic cells and its modulation by TGF beta. Cell Mol Biol (Noisy-le-grand). 1995;41:1039–49.
56. Schrauwen I, Thys M, Vanderstraeten K, Fransen E, Dieltjens N, Huyghe JR, Ealy M, Claustres M, Cremers CR, Dhooge I, Declau F, Van de Heyning P, Vincent R, Somers T, Offeciers E, Smith RJ, Van Camp G. Association of bone morphogenetic proteins with otosclerosis. J Bone Miner Res. 2008;23:507–16.
57. Lehnerdt G, Metz KA, Trellakis S, Jahnke K, Neumann A. Signaling by way of type IB and II bone morphogenetic protein receptors regulates bone formation in otospongiosis. Laryngoscope. 2007;117:812–6. Erratum in: Laryngoscope. 2007; 117:1510.
58. Lehnerdt G, Unkel C, Metz KA, Jahnke K, Neumann A. Immunohistochemical evidence of BMP-2, -4 and -7 activity in otospongiosis. Acta Otolaryngol. 2008;128:13–7.
59. Csomor P, Liktor B, Liktor B, Szekanecz Z, Sziklai I, Karosi T. Expression of bone morphogenetic protein 2, 4, 5, and 7 correlates with histological activity of otosclerotic foci. Acta Otolaryngol. 2012;132: 624–31.
60. Karosi T, Csomor P, Szalmás A, Kónya J, Petkó M, Sziklai I. Osteoprotegerin expression and sensitivity in otosclerosis with different histological activity. Eur Arch Otorhinolaryngol. 2011;268:357–65.
61. Csomor P, Sziklai I, Liktor B, Szabó L, Pytel J, Jóri J, Karosi T. Otosclerosis: disturbed balance between cell survival and apoptosis. Otol Neurotol. 2010;31:867–74.
62. Grayeli AB, Escoubet B, Bichara M, Julien N, Silve C, Friedlander G, Sterkers O, Ferrary E. Increased activity of the diastrophic dysplasia sulfate transporter in otosclerosis and its inhibition by sodium fluoride. Otol Neurotol. 2003;24:854–62.
63. Imauchi Y, Lombès M, Lainé P, Sterkers O, Ferrary E, Grayeli AB. Glucocorticoids inhibit diastrophic dysplasia sulfate transporter activity in otosclerosis by interleukin-6. Laryngoscope. 2006;116:1647–50.
64. Grayeli AB, Sterkers O, Roulleau P, Elbaz P, Ferrary E, Silve C. Parathyroid hormone-parathyroid hormone-related peptide receptor expression and function in otosclerosis. Am J Physiol. 1999;277:1005–12.
65. Fanó G, Venti-Donti G, Belia S, Paludetti G, Antonica A, Donti E, Maurizi M. PTH induces modification of transductive events in otosclerotic bone cell cultures. Cell Biochem Funct. 1993;11: 257–61.
66. Takayanagi H. Osteoimmunology: shared mechanisms and crosstalk between the immune and bone systems. Nat Rev Immunol. 2007;7:292–304.
67. Sørensen MS, Frisch T, Bretlau P. Dynamic bone studies of the labyrinthine capsule in relation to otosclerosis. Adv Otorhinolaryngol. 2007;65:53–8.
68. Frisch T, Bretlau P, Sorensen MS. Intravital microlesions in the human otic capsule. Detection, classification and pathogenetic significance revisited. ORL J Otorhinolaryngol Relat Spec. 2008;70:195–201.

69. Frisch T, Sørensen MS, Overgaard S, Bretlau P. Predilection of otosclerotic foci related to the bone turnover in the otic capsule. Acta Otolaryngol Suppl. 2000;543:111–3.
70. Wittrant Y, Theoleyre S, Chipoy C, Padrines M, Blanchard F, Heymann D, Redini F. RANKL/RANK/OPG: new therapeutic targets in bone tumours and associated osteolysis. Biochim Biophys Acta. 2004;1704:49–57.
71. Karosi T, Jókay I, Kónya J, Petkó M, Szabó LZ, Pytel J, Jóri J, Sziklai I. Activated osteoclasts with CD51/61 expression in otosclerosis. Laryngoscope. 2006;116:1478–84.
72. Ye SN, Yi ZX, Wang PY, Jiang SC. The role and significance of chondroitin sulfate in the development of otosclerosis. Laryngoscope. 1995;105:1005–9.
73. Niedermeyer HP, Becker ET, Arnold W. Expression of collagens in the otosclerotic bone. Adv Otorhinolaryngol. 2007;65:45–9.
74. Karosi T, Jokay I, Konya J, Petko M, Szabo LZ, Sziklai I. Expression of measles virus receptors in otosclerotic, non-otosclerotic and in normal stapes footplates. Eur Arch Otorhinolaryngol. 2007;264:607–13.
75. Karosi T, Szalmas A, Csomor P, Konya J, Petko M, Sziklai I. Disease-associated novel CD46 splicing variants and pathologic bone remodeling in otosclerosis. Laryngoscope. 2008;118:1669–76.
76. Moumoulidis I, Axon P, Baguley D, Reid E. A review on the genetics of otosclerosis. Clin Otolaryngol. 2007;32:239–47.
77. Norrby E, Oxman MN. Measles virus. In: Fields BN, Knipe DM, editors. Fields virology. New York: Raven; 1990. p. 1013–44.
78. Niedermeyer HP, Arnold W, Neubert WJ, Sedlmeier R. Persistent measles virus infection as a possible cause of otosclerosis: state of the art. Ear Nose Throat J. 2000;79:552–8.
79. Altermatt HJ, Gerber HA, Gaeng D, Müller C, Arnold W. Immunohistochemical findings in otosclerotic lesions. HNO. 1990;40:476–9.
80. Arnold W, Altermatt HJ, Kraft R, Pfaltz CR. Die Otosklerose, eine durch Paramyxoviren unterhaltene Entzündunsreaktion. HNO. 1989;37:236–41.
81. Arnold W, Friedmann I. Immunohistochemistry of otosclerosis. Acta Otolaryngol Suppl. 1990;470:124–8.
82. Arnold W, Busch R, Arnold A, Ritscher B, Neiss A, Niedermeyer HP. The influence of measles vaccination on the incidence of otosclerosis in Germany. Eur Arch Otorhinolaryngol. 2007;264:741–8.
83. Altermatt HJ, Gerber HA, Gaeng D, Müller C, Arnold W. Immunohistochemical findings in otosclerotic lesions. HNO. 1992;40:476–9.
84. Schrader M, Poppendieck J, Weber B. Immunohistologic findings in otosclerosis. Ann Otol Rhinol Laryngol. 1990;99:349–52.
85. McKenna MJ, Mills BG. Immunohistochemical evidence of measles virus antigens in active otosclerosis. Otolaryngol Head Neck Surg. 1989;101:415–21.
86. Lolov SR, Encheva VI, Kyurkchiev SD, Edrev GE, Kehayov IR. Antimeasles immunoglobulin G in sera of patients with otosclerosis is lower than that in healthy people. Otol Neurotol. 2001;22:766–70.
87. Karosi T, Kónya J, Petkó M, Szabó LZ, Pytel J, Jóri J, Sziklai I. Antimeasles IgG for serologic diagnosis of otosclerotic hearing loss. Laryngoscope. 2006;116:488–93.
88. McKenna MJ, Kristiansen AG, Haines J. Polymerase chain reaction amplification of a measles virus sequence from human temporal bone sections with active otosclerosis. Am J Otol. 1996;17:827–30.
89. Karosi T, Kónya J, Szabó LZ, Sziklai I. Measles virus prevalence in otosclerotic stapes footplate samples. Otol Neurotol. 2004;25:451–6.
90. Gantumur T, Niedermeyer HP, Neubert WJ, Arnold W. Molecular detection of measles virus in primary cell cultures of otosclerotic tissue. Acta Otolaryngol. 2006;126:811–6.
91. Grayeli AB, Palmer P, Tran Ba Huy P, Soudant J, Sterkers O, Lebon P, Ferrary E. No evidence of measles virus in stapes samples from patients with otosclerosis. J Clin Microbiol. 2000;38:2655–60.
92. Dhiman N, Jacobson RM, Poland GA. Measles virus receptors: SLAM and CD46. Rev Med Virol. 2004;14:217–29.
93. Erlenhofer C, Duprex WP, Rima BK, ter Meulen V, Schneider-Schaulies J. Analysis of receptor (CD46, CD150) usage by measles virus. J Gen Virol. 2002;83:1431–6.
94. Manchester M, Naniche D, Stehle T. CD46 as a measles receptor: form follows function. Virology. 2000;274:5–10.
95. Liszewski MK, Kemper C, Price JD, Atkinson JP. Emerging roles and new functions of CD46. Springer Semin Immunopathol. 2005;27:345–58.
96. Riley-Vargas RC, Gill DB, Kemper C, Liszewski MK, Atkinson JP. CD46: expanding beyond complement regulation. Trends Immunol. 2004;25:496–503.
97. Zaffran Y, Destaing O, Roux A, Ory S, Nheu T, Jurdic P, Rabourdin-Combe C, Astier AL. CD46/CD3 costimulation induces morphological changes of human T cells and activation of Vav, Rac and extracellular signal-regulated kinase mitogen–activated protein kinase. J Immunol. 2001;167:6780–5.
98. Astier A, Trescol-Biemont MC, Azocar O, Lamouille B, Rabourdin-Combe C. Cutting edge: CD46, a new costimulatory molecular for T cells that induces p120CBL and LAT phosphorylation. J Immunol. 2000;164:6091–5.
99. Kemper C, Chan AC, Green JM, Brett KA, Murphy KM, Atkinson JP. Activation of human $CD4^+$ cells with CD3 and CD46 induces a T-regulatory cell 1 phenotype. Nature. 2003;421:388–92.
100. Karp CL, Wysocka M, Wahl LM, Ahearn JM, Cuomo PJ, Sherry B, Trinchieri G, Griffin DE. Mechanism of suppression of cell-mediated immunity by measles virus. Science. 1996;273:228–31.
101. Kurita-Taniguchi M, Fukui A, Hazeki K, Hirano A, Tsuji S, Matsumoto M, Watanabe M, Ueda S, Seya T. Functional modulation of human macrophages

through CD46 (measles virus receptor): production of IL-12 p40 and nitric oxide in association with recruitment of protein-tyrosine phosphatase SHP-1 to CD46. J Immunol. 2000;165:5143–52.
102. Kawano M, Seya T, Koni I, Mabuchi H. Elevated serum levels of soluble membrane cofactor protein (CD46, MCP) in patients with systemic lupus erythematosus (SLE). Clin Exp Immunol. 1999;116: 542–6.
103. Kroshus TJ, Salerno CT, Yeh CG, Higgins PJ, Bolman 3rd RM, Dalmasso AP. A recombinant soluble chimeric complement inhibitor composed of human CD46 and CD55 reduces acute cardiac tissue injury in models of pig-to-human heart transplantation. Transplantation. 2000;69:2282–9.
104. Lanteri MB, Powell MS, Christiansen D, Li YQ, Hogarth M, Sandrin MS, McKenzie IF, Loveland BE. Inhibition of hyperacute transplant rejection by soluble proteins with the functional domains of CD46 and FcgammaRII. Transplantation. 2000;69:1128–36.
105. Avota E, Gassert E, Schneider-Saulines S. Measles virus-induced immunosuppression: from effectors to mechanisms. Med Microbiol Immunol. 2010;199: 227–37.
106. Tomek MS, Brown MR, Mani SR, Ramesh A, Srisailapathy CR, Coucke P, Zbar RI, Bell AM, McGuirt WT, Fukushima K, Willems PJ, Van Camp G, Smith RJ. Localization of a gene for otosclerosis to chromosome 15q25-q26. Hum Mol Genet. 1998;7:285–90.
107. Thys M, Van Den Bogaert K, Iliadou V, Vanderstraeten K, Dieltjens N, Schrauwen I, Chen W, Eleftheriades N, Grigoriadou M, Pauw RJ, Cremers CR, Smith RJ, Petersen MB, Van Camp G. A seventh locus for otosclerosis, OTSC7, maps to chromosome 6q13-16.1. Eur J Hum Genet. 2007;15:362–8.
108. Van Den Bogaert K, De Leenheer EM, Chen W, Lee Y, Nürnberg P, Pennings RJ, Vanderstraeten K, Thys M, Cremers CW, Smith RJ, Van Camp G. A fifth locus for otosclerosis, OTSC5, maps to chromosome 3q22-24. J Med Genet. 2004;41:450–3.
109. Van Den Bogaert K, Govaerts PJ, De Leenheer EM, Schatteman I, Verstreken M, Chen W, Declau F, Cremers CW, Van De Heyning PH, Offeciers FE, Somers T, Smith RJ, Van Camp G. Otosclerosis: a genetically heterogeneous disease involving at least three different genes. Bone. 2002;30:624–30.
110. Van Den Bogaert K, Govaerts PJ, Schatteman I, Brown MR, Caethoven G, Offeciers FE, Somers T, Declau F, Coucke P, Van de Heyning P, Smith RJ, Van Camp G. A second gene for otosclerosis, OTSC2, maps to chromosome 7q34-36. Am J Hum Genet. 2001;68:495–500.
111. Bel Hadj Ali I, Thys M, Beltaief N, Schrauwen I, Hilgert N, Vanderstraeten K, Dieltjens N, Mnif E, Hachicha S, Besbes G, Ben Arab S, Van Camp G. A new locus for otosclerosis, OTSC8, maps to the pericentromeric region of chromosome 9. Hum Genet. 2008;123:267–72.
112. Brownstein Z, Goldfarb A, Levi H, Frydman M, Avraham KB. Chromosomal mapping and phenotypic characterization of hereditary otosclerosis linked to the OTSC4 locus. Arch Otolaryngol Head Neck Surg. 2006;132:416–24.
113. McKenna MJ, Kristiansen AG, Bartley ML, Rogus JJ, Haines JL. Association of COL1A1 and otosclerosis: evidence for a shared genetic etiology with mild osteogenesis imperfecta. Am J Otol. 1998;19:604–10.
114. McKenna MJ, Nguyen-Huynh AT, Kristiansen AG. Association of otosclerosis with Sp1 binding site polymorphism in COL1A1 gene: evidence for a shared genetic etiology with osteoporosis. Otol Neurotol. 2004;25:447–50.
115. Rodríguez L, Rodríguez S, Hermida J, Frade C, Sande E, Visedo G, Martín C, Zapata C. Proposed association between the COL1A1 and COL1A2 genes and otosclerosis is not supported by a case-control study in Spain. Am J Med Genet A. 2004;128:19–22.
116. Thys M, Schrauwen I, Vanderstraeten K, Janssens K, Dieltjens N, Van Den Bogaert K, Fransen E, Chen W, Ealy M, Claustres M, Cremers CR, Dhooge I, Declau F, Claes J, Van de Heyning P, Vincent R, Somers T, Offeciers E, Smith RJ, Van Camp G. The coding polymorphism T263I in TGF-beta1 is associated with otosclerosis in two independent populations. Hum Mol Genet. 2007;16:2021–30.
117. Schrauwen I, Ealy M, Huentelman MJ, Thys M, Homer N, Vanderstraeten K, Fransen E, Corneveaux JJ, Craig DW, Claustres M, Cremers CW, Dhooge I, Van de Heyning P, Vincent R, Offeciers E, Smith RJ, Van Camp G. A genome-wide analysis identifies genetic variants in the RELN gene associated with otosclerosis. Am J Hum Genet. 2009;84:328–38.
118. Schett G, Zwerina J, David JP. The role of Wnt proteins in arthritis. Nat Clin Pract Rheumatol. 2008;4(9):473–80.
119. Diarra D, Stolina M, Polzer K, Zwerina J, Ominsky MS, Dwyer D, et al. Dickkopf-1 is a master regulator of joint remodeling. Nat Med. 2007;13:156–63.
120. Chai R, Xia A, Wang T, Jan TA, Hayashi T, Bermingham-McDonogh O, et al. Dynamic expression of Lgr5, a Wnt target gene, in the developing and mature mouse cochlea. J Assoc Res Otolaryngol. 2011;12:455–69.
121. Sienknecht UJ, Fekete DM. Mapping of Wnt, frizzled, and Wnt inhibitor gene expression domains in the avian otic primordium. J Comp Neurol. 2009;517:751–64.
122. Hawkins RD, Bashiardes S, Powder KE, Sajan SA, Bhonagiri V, Alvarado DM, et al. Large scale gene expression profiles of regenerating inner ear sensory epithelia. PLoS ONE. 2007;2, e525.
123. Matsuda M, Keino H. Roles of beta-catenin in inner ear development in rat embryos. Anat Embryol (Berl). 2000;202:39–48.
124. Hamersma H, Hofmeyr L. Too much bone: the middle ear in sclerosing bone dysplasias. Adv Otorhinolaryngol. 2007;65:61–7.

3 Preoperative Diagnosis of Otosclerosis

Tamás Karosi and István Sziklai

3.1 Introduction

Otosclerosis is a special inflammatory bone dyscrasia of the human otic capsule, which is quite difficult to diagnose preoperatively [1, 2]. However, it is a very important question from the clinical point of view, since there are several differential diagnostic problems. Furthermore, about one-third of stapes fixations can be considered as non-otosclerotic stapes ankylosis [3]. This point time, preoperative diagnosis of otosclerosis is not resolved completely. Preoperative consensus-based diagnostic protocols are also not available. It is reasonable to say that preoperative diagnostic methods and tools only focus on stapes fixation or other middle ear pathologies [4, 5]. Therefore, in the clinical nomenclature, it is recommended to use the terms of stapes fixation or stapes ankylosis for the cases with air-bone gap (ABG) and intact tympanic membranes [3]. Nevertheless, stapes surgery and precise intraoperative findings might not really modify this recommendation, because exact diagnosis of otosclerosis is still based on the histopathologic examination of the removed stapes footplates [1–3].

Furthermore, there are several other middle or inner ear disorders that must be distinguished from stapes fixations to avoid unnecessary stapes surgery or serious intraoperative complications, such as large vestibular aqueduct, enlarged cochlear canaliculi, superior semicircular canal dehiscence syndrome (SSCCD), embryonic disorders of the hearing ossicles, stapes malformations, persisting stapedial artery, or prolapsing facial nerve into the oval window niche [6–8]. These are both differential diagnostic problems and ethical-legal issues. It can be envisioned that in the future and also today, more and more rigorous legal restrictions will apply [9, 10]. This situation requires a quick reaction from ear surgeons and a rather distinct and consensus-based preoperative diagnostic protocol or recommendation from the otologic societies [9, 10]. Precise preoperative examinations may help to avoid "blind surgery," i.e., explorative tympanotomy [10]. We should accept and understand that most of the patients want to know the background of their hearing loss before signing an informed consent for stapes surgery [9].

Finally, a question arises: why is it so important to diagnose otosclerosis itself? The answer is hiding in the characteristics and consequences of the disease. Otosclerosis is a progressive disease of young patients with female dominancy. It can

T. Karosi, MD, PhD, HSc (✉)
Department of Otolaryngology and Head and Neck Surgery, B-A-Z County Hospital and University Hospital, Szentpéteri Kapu 72-76, Miskolc 3526, Hungary
e-mail: karositamas@gmail.com

I. Sziklai
Department of Otolaryngology and Head and Neck Surgery, Clinical Center, University of Debrecen, Debrecen, Hungary

I. Sziklai (ed.), *Surgery of Stapes Fixations*, DOI 10.1007/978-3-319-28576-4_3

lead to serious sensorineural hearing loss in contrast to the successful stapes surgery [1, 2]. Usually, the inflammatory bone remodeling disorder affects both ears. Female patients have serious contraindications for the usage of oral anticoncipients and also for sexual hormone substitution [11, 12]. The pregnancy and family planning is another and a rather difficult question. In conclusion, the diagnosis of otosclerosis has a great prognostic value, which can modify patient's future and quality of life in several points [11, 12].

3.2 Preoperative Diagnostic Tools

It should be established that there are no otosclerosis-specific preoperative diagnostic evaluations, which might reach enough high levels of specificity or sensitivity for the disease. However, combination of various examinations may be helpful in the differential diagnosis and can provide a rather strong clinical suspicion for otosclerosis.

Clinical diagnosis of stapes fixation is based on case history (progressive hearing loss, tinnitus, dizziness, paracusis, familial aggregation, etc.), normal otoscopic findings, negative Rinne's test, conductive and/or mixed hearing loss, type-As tympanograms, and increased resonance frequency (>1100 Hz) confirmed by multifrequency tympanometry [13, 14]. The most exact diagnosis of otosclerosis is still based on the postoperative histopathologic analysis of the removed ankylotic stapes footplates [3, 15, 16]. However, there are several limitations: most ear surgeons prefer stapedotomy or partial stapedectomy by piston technique, which are not suitable methods to obtain whole stapes footplate specimens [17]. Furthermore, in some cases of early otosclerosis, the stapes footplate is not affected by spongiotic lesions (e.g., ligament fixation), which can lead to misdiagnosis [1, 3, 12].

3.2.1 Otomicroscopy

During the physical examination, otomicroscopy has the most important role in the first medical visit. In case of otosclerosis, we can find a normal and intact tympanic membrane. Calcification of the *annulus fibrocartilaginous* or small calcified patches on the tympanic membrane are not those findings which would exclude the diagnosis of otosclerosis. In some cases, active otosclerosis might be associated with Schwartze's sign (flamingo symptom) as a consequence of hypervascularization of the promontorial mucosal lining (Fig. 3.1). It can be rarely observed, because it presumes a thin and transparent tympanic membrane [18]. This finding, however, is not specific, and its absence does not exclude existing otosclerosis.

3.2.2 Audiological Examinations

Spongiotic new bone formation in otosclerosis can result in conductive – (CHL) – and sensorineural hearing loss (SNHL) due to stapes ankylosis and pericochlear bone lesions [1, 2]. Fenestral otosclerosis is characterized by aberrant bone apposition at the *fissula ante fenestram*, which tends to grow toward the annular ligament (e.g., ligament fixation) and also the stapes footplate (stapes ankylosis) [1]. Retrofenestral otosclerosis can cause pure SNHL due to fine architectural changes in the modiolar and in the pericochlear bone (both apical and basal) resulting in decreased elasticity of the spiral ligament [1, 2, 19].

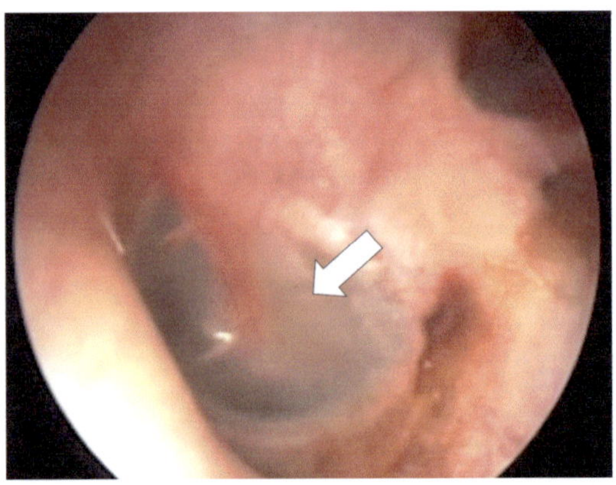

Fig. 3.1 Schwartze's sign (otomicroscopic photograph, left ear). The *white arrow* indicates the promontorial hyperemia as a consequence of hypervascularization due to the reactivated bone remodeling. It is a.k.a flamingo symptom

Complex audiologic evaluation serves as the basis of the diagnosis of CHL, mixed hearing loss (MHL), or SNHL. Subjective or objective audiological examinations, however, are not specific for otosclerosis. In contrast, they can confirm the diagnosis of stapes ankylosis or ossicular chain fixation. Nevertheless, these examinations are not suitable for the exclusion of large vestibular aqueduct or SSCCD syndrome [6]. Negative Rinne's test (C3, 1024 Hz tuning fork) on the affected ear might confirm the diagnosis of ossicular chain fixation. It is so sensitive method that a well-experienced stapes surgeon can make a decision for surgical intervention observing this phenomenon [20, 21]. However, indication for stapes surgery is based on 30 dB ABG at 1000 Hz on pure tone audiometry (PTA) [2]. The presence of ABG is very important; however, in some cases, we can find moderate or severe sensorineural component in the hearing impairment [2]. Stapes fixation is usually associated with the presence of Carhart's notch at 2000 Hz, which is a characteristic bone conduction threshold shift (Fig. 3.2). Its origin is not exactly known; however, it usually disappears after a successful stapes surgery [22]. Characteristics of ABG are also very important: toward the higher frequencies, it shows a decreasing level indicating the elastic rigidity of ossicular chain, which is sine qua non for stapes ankylosis (Fig. 3.2). PTA is seemingly a simple examination; however, it always requires adequate masking with white noise, which can be performed only by well-experienced audiologist [23]. Speech audiometry may be helpful and can provide valuable information about speech understanding, but it is not an obligatory audiologic examination in the preoperative diagnosis of otosclerosis. However, it is recommended in case of bone conduction threshold shift (MHL, SNHL) in order to exclude or confirm roll-over recruitment phenomenon [24]. On the other hand, speech audiometry is a mandatory examination, if hearing deteriorates after stapes surgery and we have to choose and fit hearing aid [24]. Preoperative tympanometry usually reveals type-As tympanograms in the affected ears. Its positivity varies between 44.18 % and 93.02 % [5, 14, 25, 26]. Stapedial reflexes show quite similar upper values, since stimulus-evoked stapedial reflex responses usually missing in the affected ears due to the immobilized stapes footplate. Multifrequency tympanometry (MFT) is much more sensitive for stapes fixation. It usually reveals 1100 Hz or higher resonance frequency in 95.34 % of the affected ears [5, 14, 25, 26].

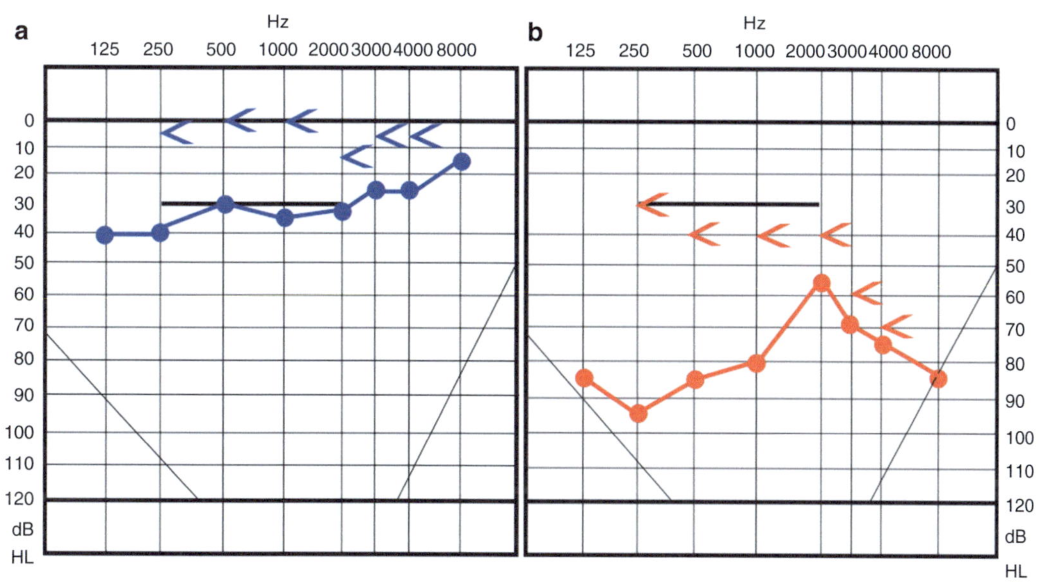

Fig. 3.2 Characteristic audiograms of clinically active and inactive (far advanced) otosclerosis. (**a**) Pure CHL, with Carhart's notch. (**b**) MHL with severe sensorineural hearing impairment

Transient-evoked otoacoustic emission (TEOAE) or distortion product otoacoustic emission (DPOAE) measurements do not help the diagnosis [5]. Stapes fixations are characterized by the absent of vestibular-evoked myogenic potential (VEMP) responses triggered by air-conduction stimuli [27]. Zhou et al. have reported that abnormally low VEMP thresholds were found in 71 of 73 ears with inner ear anomalies, such as SSCCD syndrome and enlarged vestibular aqueduct [28]. According to their results, VEMP test failed to provide accurate diagnosis in only three cases [28]. These authors have stated that VEMP test is useful during clinical evaluation of various middle and inner ear pathologies, which is characterized by higher sensitivity than tympanometry or acoustic reflexes [28]. As a final conclusion, authors have recommended the routine application of VEMP test in the differential diagnosis of these disorders to avoid unnecessary middle ear surgery for ABGs with unknown causes [28].

3.2.3 Anti-measles IgG Serology (ELISA, Enzyme-Linked Immunosorbent Assay)

Otosclerosis can be considered as a persisting measles virus infection-associated inflammatory bone remodeling disorder [29–34]. The exact role of measles virus is still not clarified in the pathogenesis of otosclerosis [1, 2, 12]. Measles virus can be an inflammatory trigger ("hit and run" hypothesis) and also can be a chronic antigen-presenting factor (autoimmune hypothesis), which lead to several immunologic or autoimmune responses in the otic capsule and also in the stapes footplate [1, 2, 12].

In 2006, Karosi et al. have performed a prospective case-controlled study including audiologic and histopathologic examinations and measles virus-specific RT-PCR (surgically removed whole stapes footplates) and anti-measles IgG serology in four patient groups [35]. Patient groups consisted of (1) histologically confirmed otosclerosis cases, (2) histologically confirmed non-otosclerosis cases, (3) patients with non-operated CHL, and (4) patients without otological disorders [35]. The serum levels of anti-measles IgG showed a statistically significant difference between the patients with virus-positive otosclerotic stapes footplates, virus-negative non-otosclerotic stapes footplates, and the control group (negative controls and patients with non-operated conductive hearing loss) [35]. It has been reported that anti-measles IgG levels were significantly lower in the sera of patients with measles virus-positive stapes footplate (median = 4 IU/ml) compared to the control groups [35]. In contrast, anti-measles IgG serum levels were normal in the controls (patients with virus-negative stapes footplates, median = 70 IU/ml; patients without hearing disorder, median = 40 IU/ml; and patients with non-operated CHL, median = 87 IU/ml) [35]. Analysis of anti-measles IgG serum levels in virus-positive stapes fixations and in virus-negative stapes fixations resulted an ROC curve (receiver operating characteristics) demonstrating diagnostic quality of anti-measles ELISA (area under curve = 0.979, $p<0.001$, standard error = 0.01) (Fig. 3.3). Authors have found that specificity and sensitivity of anti-measles serology were 90 % and 96.2 %

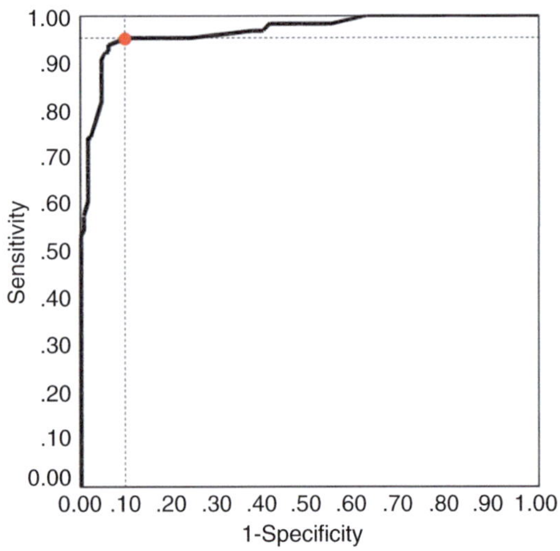

Fig. 3.3 ROC curve (receiver operating characteristics) analysis of anti-measles IgG levels of patients having measles virus-positive and virus-negative stapes footplates. Specificity and sensitivity of anti-measles ELISA were 90 % and 95.5 % by establishment of 12 IU/ml anti-measles IgG concentration in the serum as diagnostic level (area under curve = 0.968; $p<0.001$; standard error = 0.013; asymptotic 95 % confidence interval, 0.943–0.993; positive predictive value, 96.5 %; and negative predictive value, 91.1 %) [35]

with 96.5 % positive and 91.1 % negative predictive values, when anti-measles IgG serum concentration was established at 12 IU/ml as a diagnostic threshold [35]. Interestingly, low levels of anti-measles IgG in case of CHL might confirm the preoperative diagnosis of otosclerosis [35, 36].

3.2.4 High-Resolution Computed Tomography (HRCT) and Cone-Beam Computed Tomography (CBCT)

Modern imaging techniques introduced new insights into the preoperative evaluation of various osseous disorders of the human temporal bone, which have been described by several studies in otosclerosis [37–39]. High-resolution computed tomography (HRCT) scans having 0.3–0.5 mm power of resolution could detect very fine architectural changes in the otic capsule and surrounding bone structures [40] (Fig. 3.4). HRCT has also been reported as an important tool in the differential diagnosis of various middle and inner ear diseases causing conductive hearing loss, i.e., malleus head fixation, otosclerosis, and SSCCD syndrome [6, 38, 41]. Furthermore, HRCT is the main imaging method of choice in the evaluation of structural disorders in the petrous bone in cases of conductive and mixed hearing loss with normal tympanic membranes [42, 43]. HRCT is characterized by 70.5 % up to 84.2 % sensitivity levels in the detection of otosclerosis-like hypodense lesions in the otic capsule [43–45]. The specificity values of HRCT for otosclerosis, however, are not confirmed, since there are few systematic studies correlating HRCT scans to the postoperative histopathologic findings of ankylotic stapes footplates [46–48]. The diagnostic capability of HRCT is continuously developing due to the advent of more precise and higher resolution CT techniques. Preoperative detection of otosclerosis-specific hypodense lesions has great clinical significance, since it might correspond to

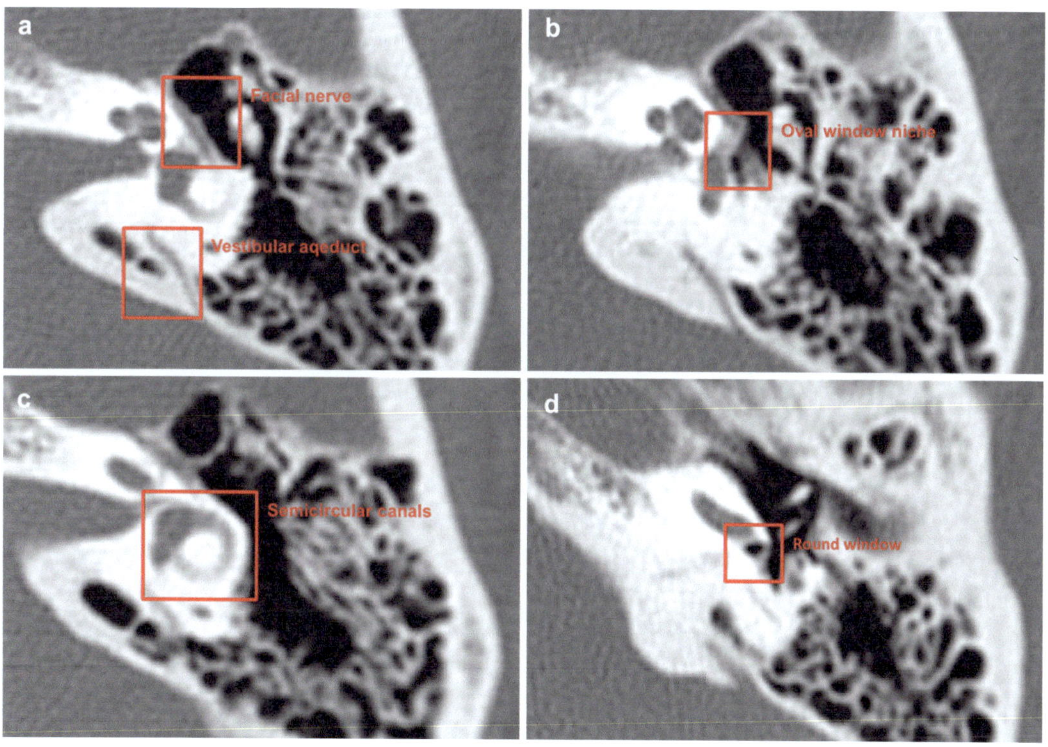

Fig. 3.4 Regions of interest (ROI) at HRCT scans. (**a**) Facial nerve and vestibular aqueduct. (**b**) Oval window niche. (**c**) Semicircular canals. (**d**) Round window

the type, severity, and progression of hearing loss [42–45]. Furthermore, it might be a real prognostic factor in the assessment of surgical success rates according to the extension and location of otosclerotic foci [45].

Cone-beam computed tomography (CBCT) is a relatively new imaging method that is widely used in the fields of endodontics and orthodontics, respectively [49, 50]. The diagnostic capability of CBCT is continuously developing due to the advent of more precise and higher resolution CT techniques and new analyzer software [49, 50]. During a CBCT scan, the single scanner and the detector rotate around the patient's head working by a cone-shaped X-ray source that results in up to 1200–2400 distinct images [49]. The specialized scanning software collects data and produces a digital volume that can be reconstructed as three-dimensional voxels containing axial-, coronal- , and sagittal dimensions [49]. The emitted X-ray dose of CBCT is about 1 % of the conventional temporal bone HRCT scans [38, 39, 50]. The scanning procedure (20–40 s) and the reconstruction time (2 min) are significantly shorter than those in HRCT [38, 50]. There are only three papers in the literature that assessed the use of CBCT in the diagnosis of otosclerosis [47, 48, 51]. In their prospective study, Redfors et al. have compared the diagnostic values of CBCT and HRCT in patients with otosclerosis, who underwent stapedectomy 30 years ago [51]. The authors have reported that CBCT is a valuable and robust imaging method for the detection of otosclerosis-like hypodense lesions in the otic capsule, which is equivalent to HRCT in many ways [51].

There is no widely accepted HRCT grading system in the assessment of severity and extension of otosclerosis in the otic capsule [41, 52–55]. *Valvassori* proposed a grading system for cochlear otosclerosis based on the size and location of hypodense lesions [41]. Later, Shin et al. reported a location-based classification for the otosclerotic foci into fenestral and pericochlear groups [43]. Pericochlear lesions were divided into two subgroups (groups 1 and 2) depending on the endosteal involvement of the cochlea [43]. Kiyomizu et al. classified the lesions into five groups as follows: *Group A*, no pathological CT findings; *Group B1*, demineralization localized in the region of the fissula ante fenestram; *Group B2*, demineralization extending toward the cochleariform process from the anterior region of the oval window; *Group B3*, extensive demineralization surrounding the cochlea; and *Group C*, thick anterior and posterior calcified plaques [52]. Rotteveel et al. introduced the terms of "*double ring effect*," "*narrowed cochlear turns*," and "*aberrant channels*" [53]. Marshall et al. and Lee et al. proposed a clinically valuable grading system for cochlear implantation in otosclerosis, which rates fenestral and cochlear lesions together (Fig. 3.5) [54, 55]. They found significant correlation between the extent of the disease and facial nerve stimulation after activation of the cochlear implant [54].

Révész et al. performed a prospective case-controlled study on 43 patients with histologically confirmed stapedial otosclerosis, who underwent unilateral stapedectomies [48]. Preoperative temporal bone CBCT and HRCT scans were performed in all cases. Both CBCT and HRCT imaging were characterized by a slice thickness of 0.4–0.625 mm and multiplanar image reconstruction. Histopathologic examination of the removed stapes footplates was performed in all cases. Findings of CBCT and HRCT were categorized according to the modified Marshall's grading system (fenestral or retrofenestral lesions). Histopathologic results were correlated to multiplanar reconstructed CBCT and HRCT scans, respectively [48]. Negative control groups for CBCT and HRCT examinations consisted of patients, who underwent CBCT imaging due to various dental disorders or HRCT analysis due to idiopathic sudden sensorineural hearing loss. Histologically active foci of otosclerosis ($n=31$, 72 %) were identified by both CBCT and HRCT in all cases with a sensitivity of 100 %. However, CBCT could not detect histologically inactive otosclerosis ($n=12$, 23 %; sensitivity=0 %) [48]. In contrast, HRCT showed inactive otosclerosis with a sensitivity of 59.3 % [48]. According to CBCT results, no retrofenestral lesions were found, and the overall sensitivity for hypodense lesions was 61.37 % [48]. They concluded that CBCT could be used only in the detection of histologically active fenestral hypodense foci of otosclerosis with high sensitivity and radiologic specificity (Figs. 3.6 and 3.7) [48].

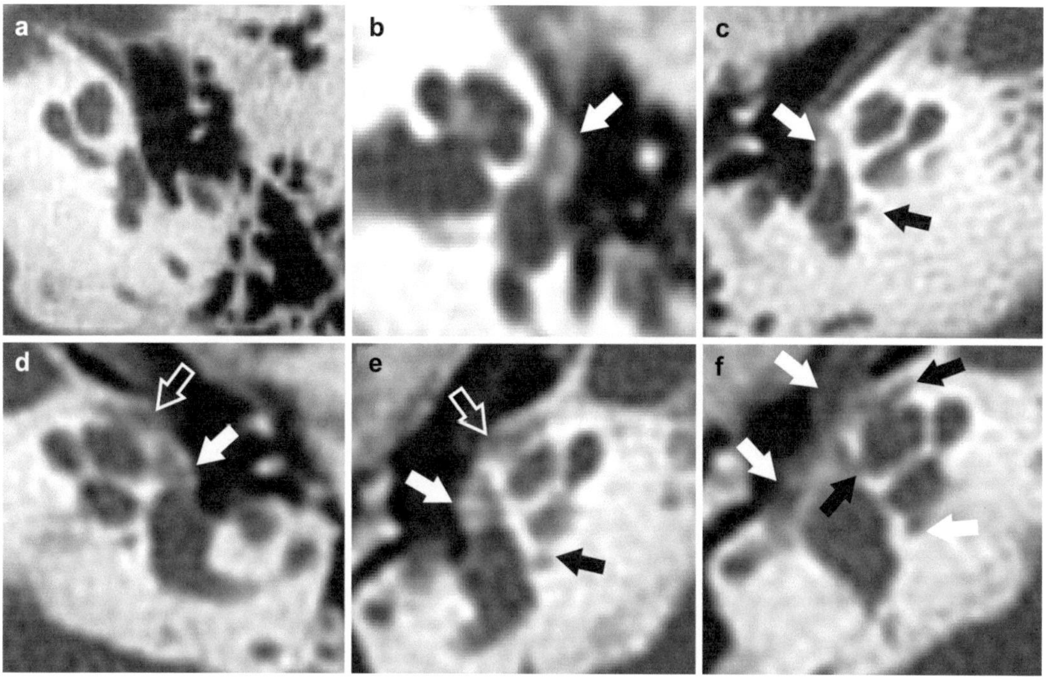

Fig. 3.5 Marshall's HRCT grading system. (**a**) *Grade 0* otosclerosis without manifest signs of hypodense lesions in the otic capsule (right ear). (**b**) *Grade 1* otosclerosis with solely fenestral lesion at the anterior pole of the stapes footplate (*white arrow*). Focus of otosclerosis has a well-defined border at the fissula ante fenestram (right ear). (**c**) *Grade 2a* otosclerosis is featured by both fenestral (*white arrow*) and basal cochlear turn lesions (*black arrow*), (left ear). (**d**) *Grade 2b* otosclerosis is presented by both fenestral (*white arrow*) and apical cochlear turn foci (*white empty arrow*), (right ear). (**e**) *Grade 2c* otosclerosis with characteristic hypodense lesions located into the anterior pole of the stapes footplate (*white arrow*), and both apical (*white empty arrow*) and basal (*black arrow*) cochlear turn of the otic capsule (left ear). (**f**) *Grade 3* otosclerosis is characterized by severe cochlear disintegration with multiple hypodense fenestral and pericochlear foci (*white arrows*). Disruption of the cochlear architecture is represented by *black arrows* (left ear) [46]

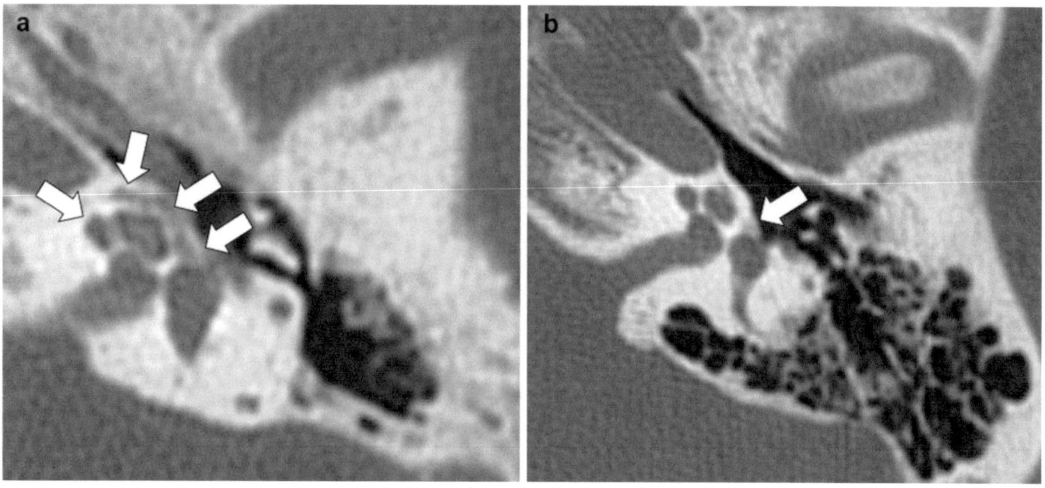

Fig. 3.6 HRCT scans of histologically confirmed otosclerosis patients. (**a**) Several hypodense lesions indicated by *white arrows* (right ear). (**b**) *White arrow* shows the thickened stapes footplate and calcified, bulky anterior pole (right ear) [46]

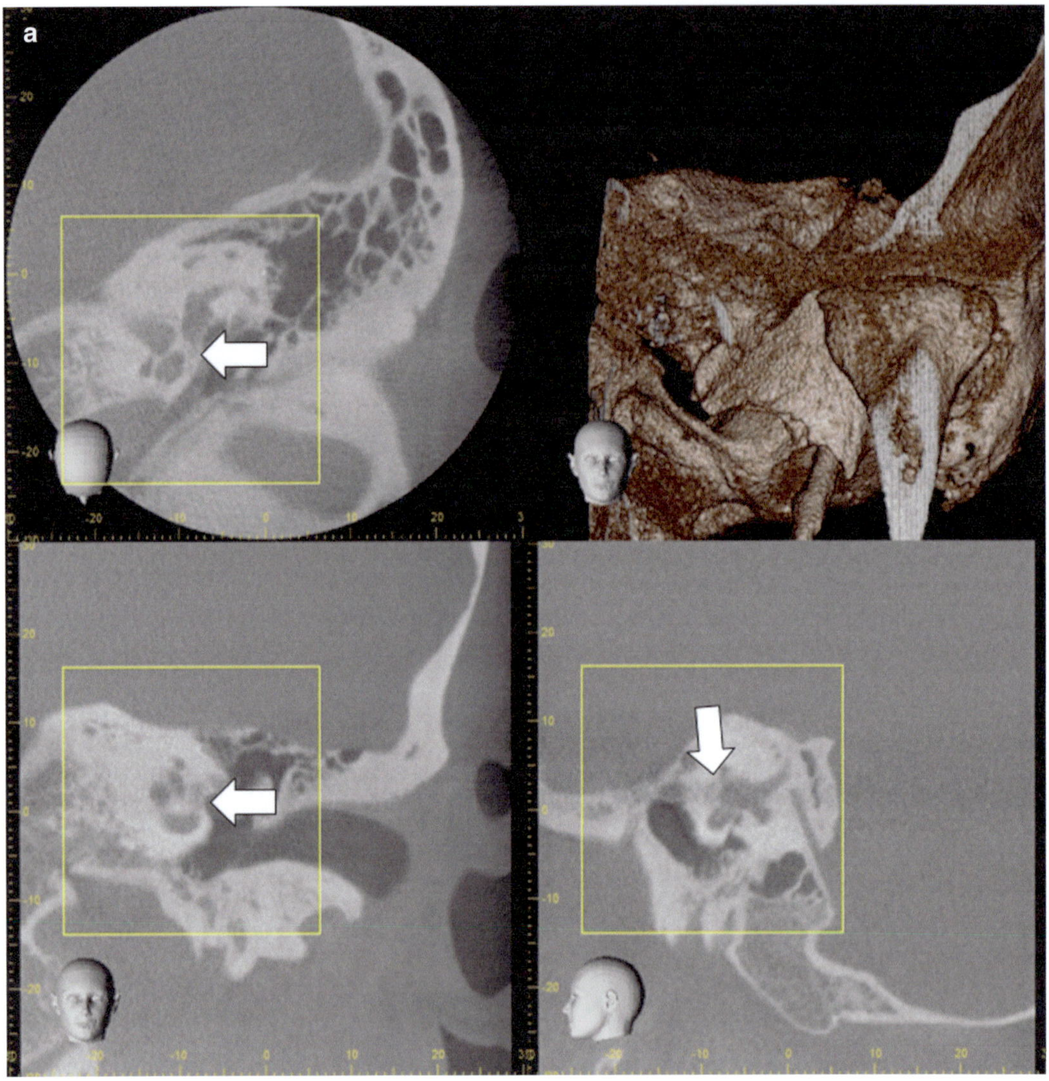

Fig. 3.7 CBCT scans of histologically confirmed otosclerosis patients. (**a**) Axial, coronal, and sagittal reconstructions of CBCT images. *White arrow* indicates a hypodense lesion at the anterior part of the oval window niche. *Yellow rectangles* show the region of interest (ROI). The *upper right* insert represents a three-dimensional reconstruction of volume rendering (left ear). (**b**) CBCT scans in histologically inactive otosclerosis (right ear). Axial, coronal, and sagittal reconstructions of CBCT images. *Grade 0* otosclerosis with no signs for hypodense lesions at the oval window niche (axial reconstruction, *white arrow*) [48]

3.3 Discussion

Otomicroscopic examination is the first and most important step in the preoperative diagnosis of stapes fixation. It is obligatory in all cases [18]. The main purpose is the exclusion of other types of middle ear disorders, which can cause CHL (chronic mesotympanic otitis, cholesteatoma, or otitis media with effusion) [18]. As we have mentioned previously, complex audiologic evaluation serves as the basis of the diagnosis of CHL, MHL, and SNHL [26]. Subjective or objective audiologic examinations, however, are not specific for otosclerosis [26]. In contrast, they can confirm the diagnosis of stapes fixation or ossicular chain fixation. Nevertheless, these

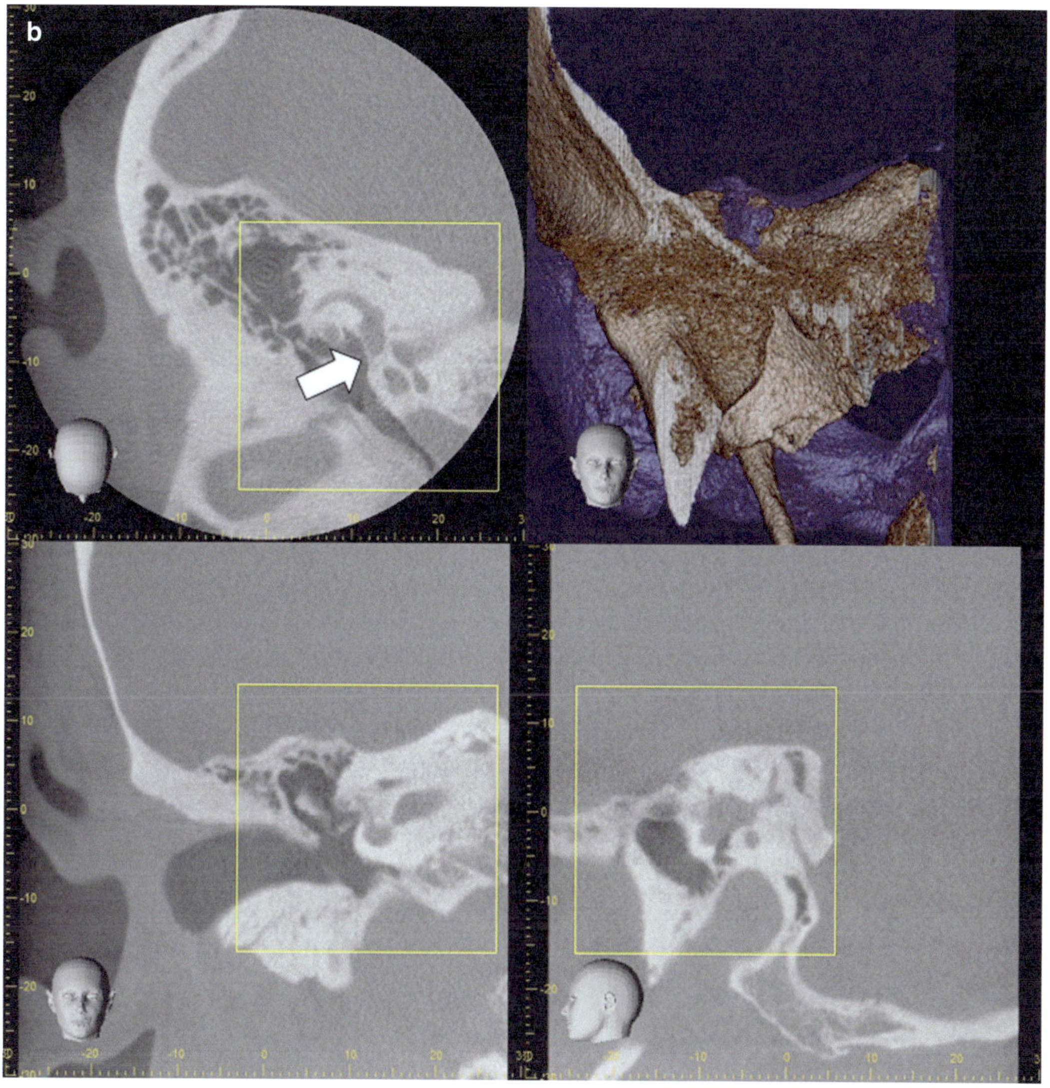

Fig. 3.7 (continued)

examinations are not suitable for the exclusion of special disorders of the inner ear that might lead to CHL [5, 14, 24, 26].

Middle ear pathologies, such as stapes fixations and otosclerosis, are characterized by the absent of VEMP responses triggered by air-conduction stimuli. VEMP seems to be a useful test during clinical evaluation of various middle and inner ear pathologies that has been reported to have higher sensitivity than tympanometry or acoustic reflexes [27, 28]. Routine application of VEMP test is recommended in the differential diagnosis of large vestibular aqueduct or SSCCD syndrome in order to avoid unnecessary middle ear surgery for ABGs with unknown causes [28]. The exact diagnostic role of VEMP test requires further systemic examinations in the future.

According to our previous results, ELISA-based anti-measles serology is highly recommended in the preoperative evaluation of patients with suspected otosclerosis [35, 36]. The humoral immune response of patients with otosclerosis should be permissive to persisting viral replication, because anti-measles IgG level is significantly decreased in these cases [35, 36]. This permissive feature of humoral immune reaction may be characteristic for otosclerosis that can be determined genetically [56, 57]. However, it is not likely that persistently infecting measles virus could directly impair the humoral immune response [56, 57]. Vaccination against measles could decrease the incidence of otosclerosis in the future; however, in spite of worldwide vaccination, measles virus circulates in the population and can induce subclinical infections in the upper respiratory tract with primary viremia [58]. Note the new measles cases in the United States [59]. Combination of decreased anti-measles IgG serum level (<12 IU/ml) and CHL with ABG at lower frequencies has a great specificity (90 %) and sensitivity (96.2 %) as a diagnostic method in the preoperative evaluation of otosclerosis [35]. This serologic method might provide the preoperative diagnosis of otosclerosis and serves as a differential diagnostic tool distinguishing non-otosclerotic stapes fixations [35]. Genetic background of the organotropism of measles virus to the otic capsule without eliciting systemic immune response remains to be elucidated [56, 57].

The most interesting question is the role and reliability of different imaging methods in the preoperative diagnosis of otosclerosis. Since, in some cases, otosclerosis might appear as the clinical picture of idiopathic sudden sensorineural hearing loss (ISSNHL), imaging is absolutely indicated in order to exclude retrocochlear lesions [60]. If we follow this train of thought, preoperative imaging is recommended in all cases of CHL with unknown origin [47, 48, 51]. Révész et al. have demonstrated various statistical associations between CBCT and HRCT scans and audiometric findings in patients with histologically confirmed otosclerosis [48]. In contrast to the relatively low number of subjects, the paper represented a comprehensive imaging and histologic study that could assess the sensitivity and specificity levels of CBCT and HRCT scans in histologically confirmed otosclerosis [48].

Sensitivity levels of HRCT scans have been reported as 70.5–84.5 % in patients with stapes fixation [44, 46]. In histologically confirmed cases, specificity levels were estimated as 100 % [46]. Redfors et al. have reported 85 % sensitivity of CBCT scans in patients with clinical otosclerosis [51]. According to our previous observations, in the group of histologically confirmed otosclerosis, CBCT showed 61.37–65.62 % overall sensitivity, which was lower, than that of previous reports [46–48]. In case of otosclerosis, HRCT showed 76.29 % overall sensitivity, which is more robust, compared to the sensitivity levels of CBCT [48]. Révész et al. have reported that CBCT was less sensitive for non-symptomatic otosclerotic foci revealing bilateral otosclerosis as 48.83 %, in contrast to the 58.14 % prevalence revealed by PTA [48]. In contrast, HRCT showed a good correspondence (55.81 %) with audiologic findings in the clinical assessment of bilateral cases [48].

As a replication of previously published data, a statistically significant association was found between the ABG averages and CBCT grades including the location of hypodense lesions in patients with histologically confirmed otosclerosis [47, 48]. This association followed an inverse function: histologically active otosclerosis with less ABG averages was characterized by positive CBCT findings; however, histologically inactive cases with larger ABG averages displayed negative CBCT scans [47, 48]. CBCT grades did not present statistically significant association with BC averages that was independent from the histologic activity of otosclerosis. On the contrary, HRCT grades (fenestral or retrofenestral) showed a statistically significant association with ABG and BC averages in the contralateral ears and also in the histologically confirmed group of stapes footplates depending on the histologic activity of otosclerosis. Regarding to HRCT findings, in case of inactive otosclerosis, the sensorineural component of hearing impairment shows a strong correlation with the severity and extension of otosclerosis. However, it cannot be confirmed by CBCT [48].

Previous studies have reported significant association between HRCT grades and the severity of preoperative ABG [42, 44, 45]. Other reports have confirmed that extension of cochlear otosclerosis estimated by HRCT correlates with the severity of SNHL [43, 46]. Similar observations, however, are not available in case of CBCT application for the preoperative diagnosis and severity assessment of otosclerosis [47, 51]. Preoperative evaluation of the extension of otosclerosis by combined application of HRCT and audiometry has a great clinical significance, since patients with far advanced cochlear otosclerosis may have benefit from cochlear implantation rather than from stapedectomy [54]. The risk of facial nerve stimulation or mispositioning of the electrode increases in this group of patients [54, 55].

The main predictors of SNHL are the endosteal involvement and cochlear wall disruption that can be well evaluated by the simple application of HRCT [46, 54, 55]. The term of *histologic otosclerosis* without hearing impairment can be explained by this phenomenon: the numbers and the location of retrofenestral otosclerotic foci are not independent predictors for the severity of SNHL [3, 15, 16]. Regarding to our previous reports, CBCT grades did not present statistically significant association with BC averages in the group of ears with different histopathologic activity of otosclerosis [48]. Therefore, CBCT seems to be an ineffective imaging method in the assessment of exact disease extension and in the evaluation of progression of SNHL [48].

In histologically inactive cases of otosclerosis, CBCT displayed 0 % sensitivity, which significantly differs from that of active otosclerosis and from that of HRCT showing 59.3 % sensitivity levels [46, 47, 51]. Inactive otosclerosis is characterized by dense and calcified osteoid substance [1, 16, 61]. Since HRCT has significantly higher sensitivity for spongiotic osseous lesions, the prevalence of sclerotic foci may be underestimated [47, 49–51]. This underestimation employing HRCT does not seriously affect the diagnosis of otosclerosis itself due to the multifocal characteristics of disease with coexisting of active and inactive foci [1, 37, 38]. CBCT is much more different: it is almost blind for retrofenestral lesions and for inactive otosclerosis [48]. In case of a solely histologically inactive fenestral otosclerotic lesion, this feature of CBCT might cause a serious diagnostic problem [6, 46, 47, 50, 51]. In the lack of histologic diagnosis, inactive fenestral otosclerosis, retrofenestral otosclerosis, and non-otosclerotic stapes fixations may occur as differential diagnostic difficulties during CBCT imaging [3, 16, 46–48]. Audiometry may be helpful in differentiation, since non-otosclerotic stapes fixations usually do not associate with SNHL [26, 37, 46, 47].

According to our previous findings, CBCT scans have very low sensitivity for retrofenestral otosclerosis [46–48]. Our previous study has concluded the following as a potential explanation for this blind phenomenon: "we do think that these are distorted findings, since our patients were not characterized by significant SNHL. These audiologic findings might reveal that our patients were not affected by cochlear otosclerosis" [47]. This conclusion must be withdrawn, since in the newest study, there were several patients suffering from significant SNHL [48]. Furthermore, HRCT scans of the individual patients revealed 13 retrofenestral and 2 round window lesions caused by otosclerosis [48].

In the light of these results, preoperative HRCT scan may serve as a valuable imaging method in the planning of stapes surgery [46]. It helps to avoid serious complications and unnecessary stapes surgeries by the detection of several abnormalities in the middle or inner ear [6, 38, 46, 47]. In contrast, Redfors et al. have reported that selected anatomic structures ($n = 16$) were clearly reconstructed by CBCT and no discrepancies were found compared to HRCT findings [51]. These results indicate that CBCT may also serve as a choice of temporal bone imaging in case of CHL with normal tympanic membranes [51]. Nevertheless, CBCT is a cheap, easy, and a rapid imaging method that is characterized by considerably lower radiation dose than HRCT [47, 49–51].

In conclusion, temporal bone HRCT is a useful imaging method in the preoperative evaluation of different types of stapes fixations and may serve as a reliable tool in the assessment of disease extension. Its sensitivity is much higher for retrofenestral lesions and for inactive otosclerosis than that of CBCT. Therefore, it can be stated that HRCT must be the first choice of temporal bone imaging. Temporal bone CBCT is a reliable imaging method in the preoperative evaluation of histologically active fenestral otosclerosis. Its overall sensitivity falls away from that of HRCT and histologic analysis, however; it continuously improves due to the introduction of more powerful analyzer software. CBCT has a doubtful correlation with hearing thresholds that depends on the histopathologic activity, the grading system, and the size of subject group. Finally, further studies are necessary to assess the precise diagnostic values of these imaging techniques.

3.4 Recommended Preoperative Diagnostic Protocol

This is a subjective, however, experience-based recommendation of the authors, which requires consensus by the national otologic societies. This recommendation considers the clinical, surgical, and also legal conditions and questions [9, 10] (Fig. 3.8).

1. Obtain a correct and precise patient's history (note the familial aggregation).
2. Perform otomicroscopy.
3. Perform subjective and objective audiologic examinations (tuning fork tests, PTA, speech audiometry, tympanometry, MFT, and VEMP).

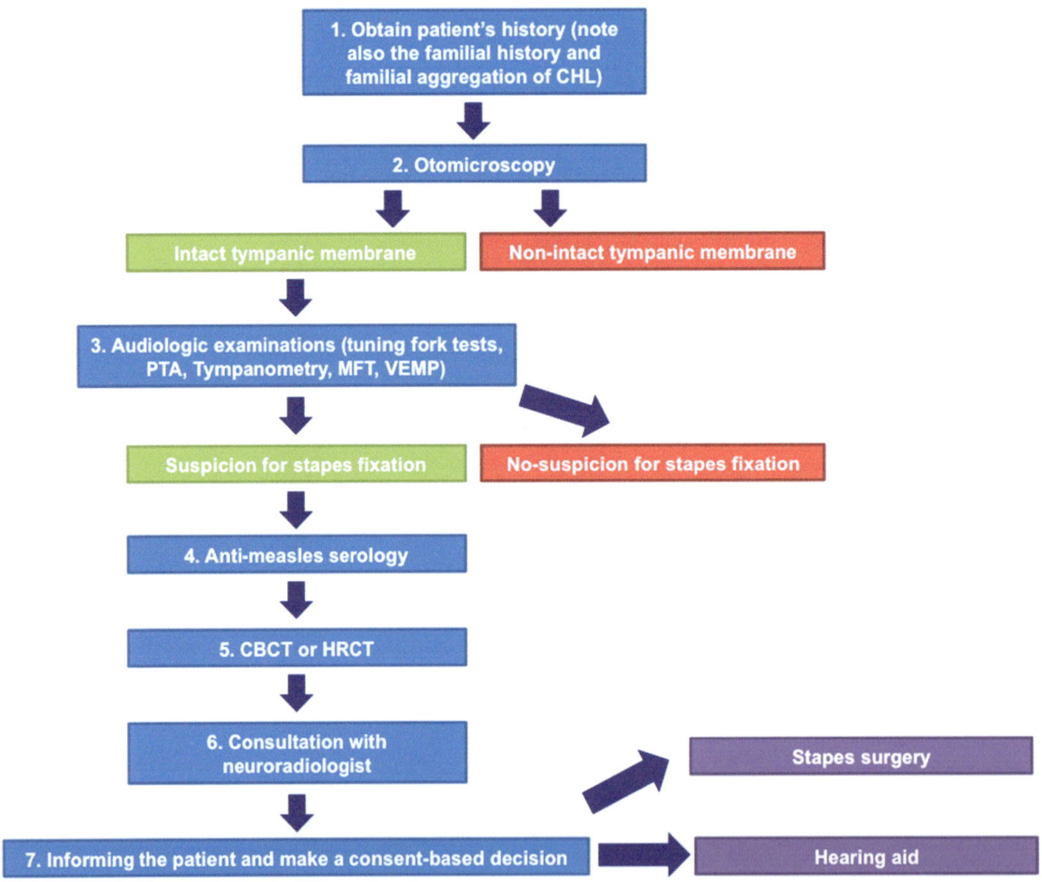

Fig. 3.8 Schematic representation of recommended diagnostic protocol for preoperative evaluation of otosclerosis

4. Analyze the anti-measles IgG serum level of the patient suspected for otosclerosis (whole blood sample without anticoagulant – ELISA).
5. Perform preoperative imaging (HRCT or CBCT) and analyze precisely the regions of interest.
6. Communicate with the radiologist/neuroradiologist.

Acknowledgments Some parts of this chapter are based on previous publications of the authors. According to scientific ethical restrictions, authors have obtained the permission for reusage of these data from Springer Scientific Publishing Group under the license numbers of 3620630353370 and 3620711246137, respectively.

References

1. Chole RA, McKenna M. Pathophysiology of otosclerosis. Otol Neurotol. 2001;22:249–57.
2. Sziklai I, Batta TJ, Karosi T. Otosclerosis: an organ-specific inflammatory disease with sensorineural hearing loss. Eur Arch Otorhinolaryngol. 2009; 266:1711–8.
3. Karosi T, Csomor P, Petkó M, Liktor B, Szabó LZ, Pytel J, Jóri J, Sziklai I. Histopathology of nonotosclerotic stapes fixations. Otol Neurotol. 2009; 30:1058–66.
4. Redfors YD, Möller C. Otosclerosis: thirty-year follow-up after surgery. Ann Otol Rhinol Laryngol. 2011;9:608–14.
5. Mantzari E, Maragoudakis P, Kandiloros D, Ferekidis E, Korres SG. The profile of otoacoustic emissions and multifrequency tympanometry in otosclerotic patients undergoing two types of stapes surgery: small fenestra and microtraumatic stapedotomy. Med Sci Monit. 2014;20:1613–20.
6. Merchant SN, Rosowski JJ, McKenna MJ. Superior semicircular canal dehiscence mimicking otosclerotic hearing loss. Adv Otorhinolaryngol. 2007;65: 137–45.
7. Moskowitz HS. Book review: review of otosclerosis diagnosis, evaluation, pathology, surgical techniques, and outcomes. Ann Otol Rhinol Laryngol. 2015;3: 250–1.
8. Sugimoto H, Ito M, Hatano M, Yoshizaki T. Persistent stapedial artery with stapes ankylosis. Auris Nasus Larynx. 2014;6:582–5.
9. Ruhl DS, Hong SS, Littlefield PD. Lessons learned in otologic surgery: 30 years of malpractice cases in the United States. Otol Neurotol. 2013;7:1173–9.
10. Blake DM, Svider PF, Carniol ET, Mauro AC, Eloy JA, Jyung RW. Malpractice in otology. Otolaryngol Head Neck Surg. 2013;4:554–61.
11. Liktor B, Szekanecz Z, Batta TJ, Sziklai I, Karosi T. Perspectives of pharmacological treatment in otosclerosis. Eur Arch Otorhinolaryngol. 2013;3:793–804.
12. Karosi T, Sziklai I. Etiopathogenesis of otosclerosis. Eur Arch Otorhinolaryngol. 2010;9:1337–49.
13. Sanford CA, Schooling T, Frymark T. Determining the presence or absence of middle ear disorders: an evidence-based systematic review on the diagnostic accuracy of selected assessment instruments. Am J Audiol. 2012;2:251–68.
14. Shahnaz N, Bork K, Polka L, Longridge N, Bell D, Westerberg BD. Energy reflectance and tympanometry in normal and otosclerotic ears. Ear Hear. 2009;2:219–33.
15. Declau F, van Spaendonck M, Timmermans JP, Michaels L, Liang J, Qiu JP, van de Heyning P. Prevalence of histologic otosclerosis: an unbiased temporal bone study in Caucasians. Adv Otorhinolaryngol. 2007;65:6–16.
16. Iyer PV, Gristwood RE. Histopathology of the stapes in otosclerosis. Pathology. 1984;16:30–8.
17. Kamalski DM, Wegner I, Tange RA, Vincent R, Stegeman I, van der Heijden GJ, Grolman W. Outcomes of different laser types in laser-assisted stapedotomy: a systematic review. Otol Neurotol. 2014;6:1046–51.
18. Nakashima T, Sone M, Fujii H, Teranishi M, Yamamoto H, Otake H, Sugiura M, Naganawa S. Blood flow to the promontory in cochlear otosclerosis. Clin Otolaryngol. 2006;2:110–5.
19. Sellari-Franceschini S, Ravecca F, De Vito A, Berrettini S. Progressive sensorineural hearing loss in cochlear otosclerosis. Acta Otorhinolaryngol Ital. 1998;18:59–65.
20. MacKechnie CA, Greenberg JJ, Gerkin RC, McCall AA, Hirsch BE, Durrant JD, Raz Y. Rinne revisited: steel versus aluminum tuning forks. Otolaryngol Head Neck Surg. 2013;6:907–13.
21. Gordon MA, Silverstein H, Willcox TO, Rosenberg SI. A reevaluation of the 512-Hz Rinne tuning fork test as a patient selection criterion for laser stapedotomy. Am J Otol. 1998;6:712–7.
22. Kashio A, Ito K, Kakigi A, Karino S, Iwasaki S, Sakamoto T, Yasui T, Suzuki M, Yamasoba T. Carhart notch 2-kHz bone conduction threshold dip: a nondefinitive predictor of stapes fixation in conductive hearing loss with normal tympanic membrane. Arch Otolaryngol Head Neck Surg. 2011;3:236–40.
23. Miller MH. How to eliminate air-bone gaps audiometrically: use too much masking. Ear Nose Throat J. 2008;5:273–6.
24. Abdelghaffar H, Fakhry S, Fawzy T. Aided air conduction threshold as a predictor of cochlear reserve in otosclerosis patients. ORL J Otorhinolaryngol Relat Spec. 2010;1:12–5.
25. Miani C, Bergamin AM, Barotti A, Isola M. Multifrequency multicomponent tympanometry in normal and otosclerotic ears. Scand Audiol. 2000;4:225–37.

26. Probst R. Audiological evaluation of patients with otosclerosis. Adv Otorhinolaryngol. 2007;65:119–26.
27. Tramontani O, Gkoritsa E, Ferekidis E, Korres SG. Contribution of Vestibular-Evoked Myogenic Potential (VEMP) testing in the assessment and the differential diagnosis of otosclerosis. Med Sci Monit. 2014;20:205–13.
28. Zhou G, Poe D, Gopen Q. Clinical use of vestibular evoked myogenic potentials in the evaluation of patients with air-bone gaps. Otol Neurotol. 2012;8:1368–74.
29. Arnold W, Niedermeyer HP, Lehn N, Neubert W, Höfler H. Measles virus in otosclerosis and the specific immune response of the inner ear. Acta Otolaryngol. 1996;116:705–9.
30. Niedermeyer HP, Arnold W. Otosclerosis: a measles virus associated inflammatory disease. Acta Otolaryngol. 1995;115:300–3.
31. Karosi T, Kónya J, Petkó M, Sziklai I. Histologic otosclerosis is associated with the presence of measles virus in the stapes footplate. Otol Neurotol. 2005;26:1128–33.
32. Arnold W, Friedmann I. Otosclerosis – an inflammatory disease of the otic capsule of viral aetiology? J Laryngol Otol. 1988;102:865–71.
33. McKenna MJ, Mills BG. Ultrastructural and immunohistochemical evidence of measles virus in active otosclerosis. Acta Otolaryngol Suppl. 1990;470:130–40.
34. Niedermeyer HP, Arnold W, Schuster M, Baumann C, Kramer J, Neubert WJ, Sedlmeier R. Persistent measles virus infection and otosclerosis. Ann Otol Rhinol Laryngol. 2001;110:897–903.
35. Karosi T, Kónya J, Petkó M, Szabó LZ, Pytel J, Jóri J, Sziklai I. Antimeasles IgG for serologic diagnosis of otosclerotic hearing loss. Laryngoscope. 2006;116:488–93.
36. Lolov SR, Encheva VI, Kyurkchiev SD, Edrev GE, Kehayov IR. Antimeasles immunoglobulin G in sera of patients with otosclerosis is lower than that in healthy people. Otol Neurotol. 2001;22:766–70.
37. Mafee MF, Henrikson GC, Deitch RL, Norouzi P, Kumar A, Kriz R, Valvassori GE. Use of CT in stapedial otosclerosis. Radiology. 1985;156:709–14.
38. Shaffer KA, Haughton VM, Wilson CR. High resolution computed tomography of the temporal bone. Radiology. 1980;134:409–14.
39. Grayeli AB, Yrieix CS, Imauchi Y, Cyna-Gorse F, Ferrary E, Sterkers O. Temporal bone density measurements using CT in otosclerosis. Acta Otolaryngol. 2004;124:1136–40.
40. Lagleyre S, Sorrentino T, Calmels MN, Shin YJ, Escudé B, Deguine O, Fraysse B. Reliability of high-resolution CT scan in diagnosis of otosclerosis. Otol Neurotol. 2009;30:1152–9.
41. Valvassori GE. Imaging of otosclerosis. Otolaryngol Clin N Am. 1993;26:359–71.
42. Naumann IC, Porcellini B, Fisch U. Otosclerosis: incidence of positive findings on high-resolution computed tomography and their correlation to audiological test data. Ann Otol Rhinol Laryngol. 2005;114:709–16.
43. Shin YJ, Fraysse B, Deguine O, Cognard C, Charlet JP, Sévely A. Sensorineural hearing loss and otosclerosis: a clinical and radiologic survey of 437 cases. Acta Otolaryngol. 2001;121:200–4.
44. Marx M, Lagleyre S, Escudé B, Demeslay J, Elhadi T, Deguine O, Fraysse B. Correlations between CT scan findings and hearing thresholds in otosclerosis. Acta Otolaryngol. 2011;131:351–7.
45. Wycherly BJ, Berkowitz F, Noone AM, Kim HJ. Computed tomography and otosclerosis: a practical method to correlate the sites affected to hearing loss. Ann Otol Rhinol Laryngol. 2010;119:789–94.
46. Karosi T, Csomor P, Sziklai I. The value of HRCT in stapes fixations corresponding to hearing thresholds and histologic findings. Otol Neurotol. 2012;8:1300–7.
47. Liktor B, Révész P, Csomor P, Gerlinger I, Sziklai I, Karosi T. Diagnostic value of cone-beam CT in histologically confirmed otosclerosis. Eur Arch Otorhinolaryngol. 2014;8:2131–8.
48. Révész P, Liktor B, Liktor B, Sziklai I, Gerlinger I, Karosi T. Comparative analysis of preoperative diagnostic values of HRCT and CBCT in patients with histologically diagnosed otosclerotic stapes footplates. Eur Arch Otorhinolaryngol. 2016 Jan;273(1):63–72. http://www.ncbi.nlm.nih.gov/pubmed/25559466 doi: 10.1007/s00405-015-3490-3. Epub 2015 Jan 6. PMID: 25559466.
49. Patel S, Dawood A, Ford TP, Whaites E. The potential applications of cone beam computed tomography in the management of endodontic problems. Int Endod J. 2007;40:818–30.
50. Small BW. Cone beam computed tomography. Gen Dent. 2007;55:179–81.
51. Redfors YD, Gröndahl HG, Hellgren J, Lindfors N, Nilsson I, Möller C. Otosclerosis: anatomy and pathology in the temporal bone assessed by multi-slice and cone-beam CT. Otol Neurotol. 2012;33:922–7.
52. Kiyomizu K, Tono T, Yang D, Haruta A, Kodama T, Komune S. Correlation of CT analysis and audiometry in Japanese otosclerosis. Auris Nasus Larynx. 2004;31:125–9.
53. Rotteveel LJ, Proops DW, Ramsden RT, Saeed SR, van Olphen AF, Mylanus EA. Cochlear implantation in 53 patients with otosclerosis: demographics, computed tomographic scanning, surgery, and complications. Otol Neurotol. 2004;25:943–52.
54. Marshall AH, Fanning N, Symons S, Shipp D, Chen JM, Nedzelski JM. Cochlear implantation in cochlear otosclerosis. Laryngoscope. 2005;115:1728–33.
55. Lee TC, Aviv RI, Chen JM, Nedzelski JM, Fox AJ, Symons SP. CT grading of otosclerosis. Am J Neuroradiol. 2009;30:1435–9.
56. Karosi T, Jokay I, Konya J, Petko M, Szabo LZ, Sziklai I. Expression of measles virus receptors in otosclerotic, non-otosclerotic and in normal stapes footplates. Eur Arch Otorhinolaryngol. 2007;264:607–13.
57. Karosi T, Szalmas A, Csomor P, Konya J, Petko M, Sziklai I. Disease-associated novel CD46 splicing

variants and pathologic bone remodeling in otosclerosis. Laryngoscope. 2008;118:1669–76.
58. Arnold W, Busch R, Arnold A, Ritscher B, Neiss A, Niedermeyer HP. The influence of measles vaccination on the incidence of otosclerosis in Germany. Eur Arch Otorhinolaryngol. 2007;264:741–8.
59. Liu F, Enanoria WT, Zipprich J, Blumberg S, Harriman K, Ackley SF, Wheaton WD, Allpress JL, Porco TC. The role of vaccination coverage, individual behaviors, and the public health response in the control of measles epidemics: an agent-based simulation for California. BMC Public Health. 2015;1:447.
60. Schuknecht HF. Myths in neurotology. Am J Otol. 1992;2:124–6.
61. Parahy C, Linthicum Jr FH. Otosclerosis and otospongiosis: clinical and histological comparisons. Laryngoscope. 1984;94:508–12.

4 Stapedectomy

István Sziklai

4.1 Aims of Surgical Intervention in Stapes Fixation

Stapes fixation caused conductive hearing loss can be restored by mechanical reconstruction of the mobility of the sound-transmitting ossicular system. This can be achieved by mobilization of the stapes footplate [24], by removal of the stapes and replacing by a prosthesis [12], or by removal of the stapes superstructure and connecting the vestibule to the lenticular process of the incus by a prosthesis [13, 27]. Different surgical techniques differ from each other in many respects and exhibit the evolution of the surgical treatment in stapes fixations. The first stapedectomies were performed in the 1950s [10]. Shea was, however, the first who reported about good and stable hearing results after stapedectomy [28]. Shea covered the oval window with vein graft and replaced the stapes superstructure by a polyethylene tube. Many surgeons used this technique for many years successfully, and they obtained long-standing good hearing results. Approaching the middle ear cavity was changed from retroauricular incision toward endaural and then endomeatal incision. These changes optimized the visualization of the oval window niche. Meanwhile, opening the vestibule through the fixed stapes footplate moved from extracting the stapes footplate toward fenestration of the footplate by lasers of different types (argon, CO2, KTP, erbium) [5, 11, 14, 15, 35]. The surgical harm and risk of intraoperative complications could be decreased by these changes. Sealing the vestibule by different types of grafting materials, e.g., vein, fascia, connective tissue, fat, and gelfoam, leads to calibrating the predictable hearing improvement gain more precisely. Aiming to obtain the best possible hearing result, postoperatively, the design and substance of the stapes prosthesis and the piston also followed important changes from polyethylene toward biocompatible ceramics, Teflon wire, gold, titanium, and stainless steel [19, 30]. The size of the opening into the vestibule is decreased from total stapedectomy to partial stapedectomy and then to a hole of different size between 0.4 and 0.8 mm (stapedotomy) [23]. This initiated a negotiation on the preferable surgical technique to achieve the best hearing result. The controversial issues related to stapedectomy (total removal of the stapes footplate) or stapedotomy (making only a hole in the footplate) are hearing in the speech frequencies (0.5 to 1–2 kHz), hearing in the high frequencies (4 and 8 kHz), stability of hearing, postoperative vertigo/unsteadiness, and tinnitus. In an important report on this issue,

---

Electronic supplementary material The online version of this chapter (doi:10.1007/978-3-319-28576-4_4) contains supplementary material, which is available to authorized users.

I. Sziklai
Department of Otolaryngology and Head and Neck Surgery, Clinical Center, University of Debrecen, Debrecen, Hungary
e-mail: isziklai@med.unideb.hu

I. Sziklai (ed.), *Surgery of Stapes Fixations*, DOI 10.1007/978-3-319-28576-4_4

Rizer and Lippy compared the hearing results after total stapedectomy, partial stapedectomy, and stapedotomy [23]. He found the best, although not significantly the best, hearing results in each frequency after total stapedectomy.

Beside the primary goal of eliminating conductive hearing loss, another goal can be improving the sensorineural loss in a mixed type hearing loss. The stapes fixation related bone conduction threshold elevation below 4 kHz is a well-known audiological consequence of the restriction in the basilar membrane vibration characteristics which has already been suspected by Carhart and Hayes in the late 1940s [4]. The consequence is that abolishing the stapes fixation results in a bone conduction threshold improvement after stapedectomy [1].

In the property of the cochlear implantation, the profound deafness in otosclerosis, the unsuccessful outcome of stapes surgery, or postoperative deafness enters in our view very differently. However, cochlear implantation is not able to provide with such high-fidelity speech and music sound presentation like physiological hearing or hearing with a hearing aid. Stapedectomy can aim to improve the hearing in profound mixed hearing loss cases to a serviceable level by hearing aid [8].

4.2 Preoperative Diagnostics

This topic is overviewed in Chap. 3 in details. Preoperative examinations before stapedectomy, however, should try to clarify the following possible abnormalities in the surgical field. Some of them may contraindicate stapedectomy.

- The fixation of the stapes is otosclerotic or non-otosclerotic?
- It can be clarified by determining the anti-measles IgG level in the serum of the conductive hearing loss patient [17]. Lower than 10 IU/ml serum concentration suggests otosclerosis highly probable. Temporal bone CT scanning may also exhibit active otosclerosis by perilabyrinthine bone resorption. The rational of clarifying the nature of the stapes fixation preoperatively is as follow. In case of otosclerosis, the heavy fixation of the footplate and the thickened and highly vascularized mucosal lining in the oval window niche decrease the risk of a floating footplate. Even small fragments are fixed well by the attached mucosal lining. In case of non-otosclerotic fixations, the interface between the stapes footplate and the oval window (annular ligament) is smooth and allows some mobility when the friction by the bulky excess bone is decreased by removal of some part of the stapes. This may easily lead to floating footplate.
- Intact or dehiscent facial nerve canal. It may decide whether stapedectomy can be performed or not. Stapedotomy should rather be considered in the case of overhanging facial nerve which covers partly or mostly the oval window.
- Large vestibular aqueduct, Mondini dysplasia can also exclude the possibility of stapedectomy because of gusher. A trial of stapedotomy may be attempted. Some special manipulations can result in saving the hearing simultaneously with closure of the perilymph/CSF leak.
- Obliterative otosclerosis established by imaging can also exclude stapedectomy. Using microdrill and making a hole in the oval window niche and partly on the promontory at the middle segment of the niche are preferable [25].
- Ossified round window is contraindication for stapedectomy/stapedotomy. Better results can be obtained by BAHA even in single-sided deafness.

4.3 Indications and Contraindications for Exploratory Tympanotomy in the Suspicion of Stapes Fixation

4.3.1 Indications

Conductive hearing loss behind intact tympanic membrane with negative Rinne tuning fork test at 512 Hz arises consideration of surgery to improve the hearing. An anti-measles IgG seronegativity confirms the presence of an otosclerotic stapes fixation caused conductive hearing loss [17]. Ossicular chain fixation of any etiology is confirmed by a low peak tympanogram with normal middle ear pressure and with non-elicitable stapedius reflex. Mixed hearing loss which is not serviceable by hearing aid fitting indicates exploration of the middle ear cavity. Stapedectomy may be attempted for achieving such level of hearing threshold which is serviceable by hearing aid.

4.3.2 Contraindications

An only hearing ear with serviceable hearing should not be operated on. A BAHA fitting will provide satisfactory hearing for the patient without jeopardizing a total hearing loss. Chronic suppurative otitis media first should be eradicated, and as a second step surgery stapedectomy can be attempted. Infection in the external auditory meatus should be managed similarly. Meniere's disease combined with conductive hearing loss due to stapes fixation is a special situation. The saccule is distended in endolymphatic hydrops and easy to puncture it which leads to sensorineural hearing loss. Large vestibular aqueduct and X chromosome-linked gusher are contraindications, but stapedotomy may be attempted.

4.4 Stapedectomy

Stapedectomy is criticized for a long time because of the large opening of the vestibule made in the oval window as potential harm for the membranous labyrinth. Also, from the beginning of its application, a postoperative high-frequency sensorineural hearing loss development due to stapedectomy turned out as a possible outcome. This is debated by many surgeons (this question is highlighted in Chap. 12). The high-frequency loss can be due to surgical manipulation inside the vestibule and rather more to suction in the oval window after opening the vestibule. The bone conduction loss at 4 kHz after stapedectomy, however, doesn't exceed 3 dB when compared to the preoperative audiograms in a comprehensive study [31]. Furthermore, Arnold et al. reported [1] that the bone conduction hearing loss at 2 and 4 kHz after stapedectomy is caused by the mechanical properties of the inserted prosthesis rather than by the total removal of the stapes footplate.

Although the technical baseline for stapedectomy is universal: removal of the stapes fully or partly and replacing it by a prosthesis for hearing restoration, the diversity of different stapedectomy techniques is attributed to differences in several surgical solutions. These are the followings:

- Surgical approach to the middle ear cavity
- Type of prosthesis used for reconstruction (xenografts or autologous cortical bone columella [2]) of the ossicular chain
- Saving or sacrificing the tendon of the stapedius muscle
- Saving the posterior crus of the stapes
- Overlaying the oval window by connective tissue
- Respecting the chorda tympani
- Steps and order of surgical manipulations

4.4.1 Patient Positioning on the Operating Table

The patient is in supine position on the table, and it should facilitate the appropriate exposure to the surgeon (Fig. 4.1). Cutting hair may not be necessary except if side whiskers in males decrease the achievement for endaural incision.

Either a self-retaining speculum can be used in combination with a head resting fixation or an assistant may position the head of the patient in the required setting. A preferable view of the surgical field with good illumination to the pyramidal eminence and posterior half of the stapes footplate can be obtained by rotating the table toward the surgeon after the tympanomeatal flap is elevated.

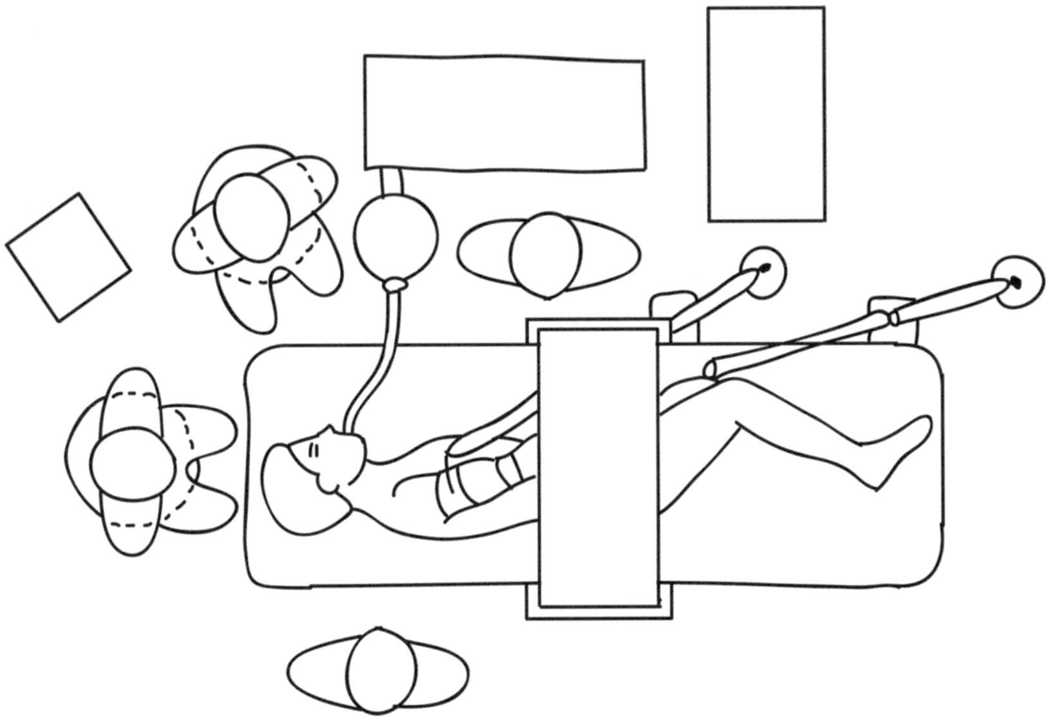

Fig. 4.1 Position of the patient on the operating table during stapes surgery. The surgeon, the assistant, and the anesthesiologist are around the head of the patient. The instrumenting nurse is on the left-hand side of the patient

4.4.2 Anesthesia

Both local anesthesia and general anesthesia can be performed. Local anesthesia is helpful to control the satisfaction of the patients with hearing level obtained by the surgery. Stapedectomy has somewhat higher risk for postoperative disequilibrium or vertigo. This is due to the close vicinity of the saccule to the stapes footplate anteriorly. During extraction of the footplate, the saccule may be damaged causing vestibular symptoms. Removal of the stapes footplate can induce vertigo, and the patient on the operating table may carry on a prompt head movement that can lead to unwanted surgical pitfalls as the surgeon is still manipulating in the middle ear cavity. Special cases (e.g., panic reaction tendency) also need general anesthesia. Local anesthesia is introduced by 2 % lidocaine with 0.001 % epinephrine. This should provide with a bloodless surgical field which is essential in stapes surgery. Infiltration of the external auditory meatus by lidocaine/epinephrine is also suggested in general anesthesia to ensure the necessary bloodless surgical field.

4.4.3 Endaural Approach (Fig. 4.2)

The skin incision begins anterior to the pinna at about 1.5–2 cm upward to the tragus and introduced into the auricle between the cartilages of the crus of helix and the tragus. The incision then continues behind the orifice of the external auditory meatus and allows elevation of the meatal skin from the bony posterior external auditory meatus superiorly and posteriorly. Self-retaining retractor is adjusted, and another retractor is positioned perpendicular to the first one providing with enough space for surgical manipulations. Care should be taken to avoid injury to the cartilaginous auricle. This causes bleeding which may result in perichondritis and cosmetically gives poor healing result. Temporal muscle aponeurosis (commonly called fascia) can be harvested for sealing the oval window or reconstructing meatal

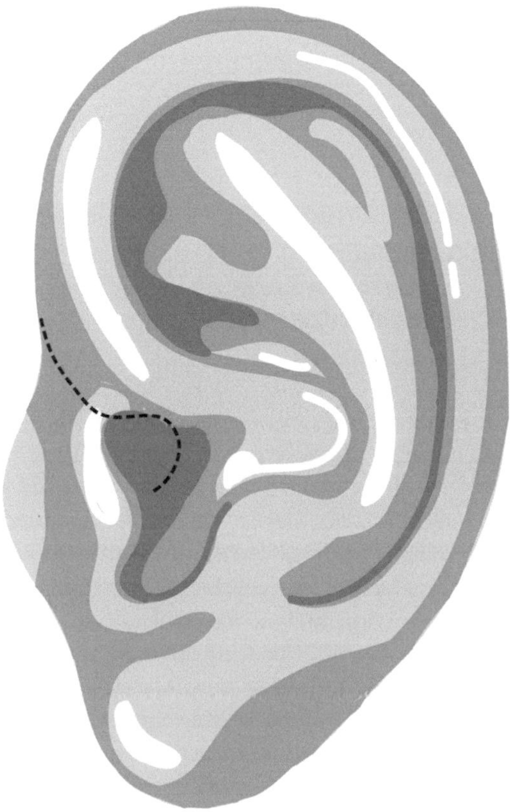

Fig. 4.2 Skin incision (*dotted line*) during the endaural approach

skin/tympanic membrane injuries if necessary. The meatal skin should be carefully, bluntly elevated from the suprameatal spine by a periosteal elevator. The spine is multiple sometimes and can be difficult to prepare the skin without tearing it. The fibrocartilaginous annulus is elevated from its bony groove by a needle and circumferentially pulled upward until the notch of Rivinus and downward in integrity with the tympanic membrane.

Exostosis can complicate the elevation of the meatal skin. They exhibit high variability of individual appearance and can lead to tears on the tympanomeatal flap. Tympanic membrane perforation or dehiscent meatal skin should be reconstructed by temporal fascia. Approaching the fibrous annulus of the drum, a needle helps to tease off it at its upper segment, and then the annulus can be separated from the groove by an elevator, downward.

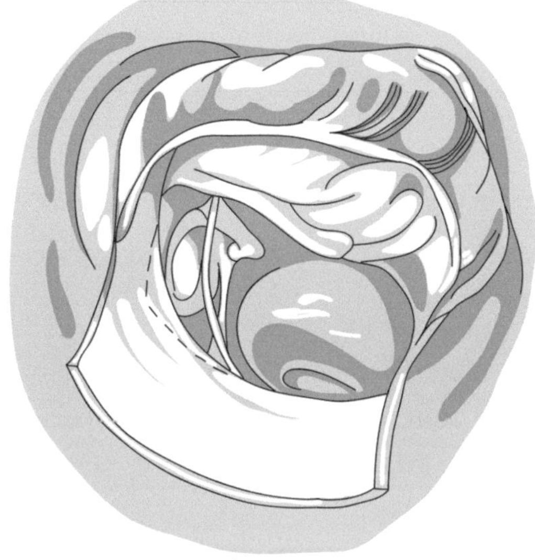

Fig. 4.3 Skin incision in an endomeatal approach

4.4.4 Endomeatal Approach (Fig. 4.3)

Incision in the meatal skin is performed from 12 to 6 o'clock direction after proper infiltration by lidocaine with epinephrine. The incision is made approximately 1 cm from the tympanic membrane (Fig. 4.3). The skin is elevated together with the periosteum medially with a raspatorium until the fibrous annulus of the tympanic membrane. The annulus is displaced anteriorly from its groove from upward to downward direction.

4.4.5 **Scutoplasty** (Video 4.1 and Fig. 4.4)

Micro-chisel is an appropriate device to take away the overhanging scutum for visualizing the incudostapedial joint. Disconnected bone pieces should be removed because remnants induce connective tissue reaction with formation of tumor-like space occupying mucosal thickening. Drilling by diamond burr can prevent damage to the chorda tympani, but the bone dust induces again mucosal proliferation that may fix the ossicular chain causing conductive hearing loss. The exact positioning of the chisel to avoid incus

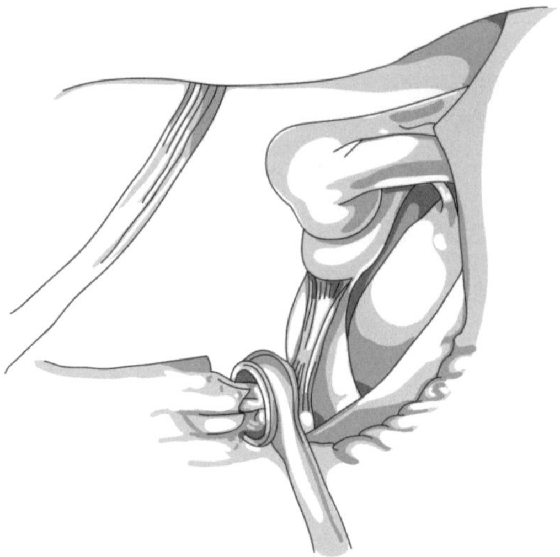

Fig. 4.4 Scutoplasty to expose the pyramidal eminence and the full oval window niche

subluxation is centered to the incudostapedial joint, and the chisel profile shouldn't exceed 4 mm. The bone pieces should be dislocated first by a needle and then can be removed by the suction tube or by a crocodile micro ear forceps. Bigger block of chiseled bone is carefully removed after separating the chorda tympani from it, first. Good view of the oval window niche means that the pyramidal eminence can be seen. Enlarging the dehiscence on the scutum may be precisely adjusted to the expectation by curettage. The surgical field is bordered in the middle ear by the round window down, the facial nerve canal superiorly, and the handle of the malleus anteriorly. Explorative tympanotomy can be finished at this point because the middle ear diseases which can potentially cause conductive hearing loss with intact tympanic membrane and normal middle ear pressure can already be established. These diseases are the followings:

1. Tympanosclerosis fixing the ossicles
2. Stapes fixation
3. Malleus fixation
4. Necrosis of the lenticular process of the incus
5. Fusion of the ossicles
6. Congenital cholesteatoma in the oval window niche
7. Facial nerve schwannoma
8. Overhanging facial nerve due to widely dehiscent fallopian canal
9. Calcification of the malleolar ligaments
10. Bony obliteration of the round window

4.4.6 Mobility of the Ossicular Chain and Anatomy of the Round Window (Video 4.2)

An important step intraoperatively is to control the mobility of the ossicular chain. First, the mobility of the stapes is checked. Its immobility demonstrates the stapes fixation. The slight movement of the incus can be provoked by a needle. Large amplitude movements should not be evoked avoiding injury to the organ of Corti/basilar membrane unit. Checking the mobility of the malleus is the following step. Malleus fixation results in failure in the hearing improvement in spite of the properly performed stapedectomy. Blue discoloration in the middle third of the footplate can be seen when the bony fixation is localized to the anterior pole of the stapes. Missing blue color denotes an obliterative thickening of the footplate.

The round window is examined to exclude ossification. Usually the endaural approach gives enough view to bring the round window into the field. When the round window cannot be achieved by microscope, an endoscope of 0° or 30° can be used. The round window morphology is highly variable case by case. Its surrounding bony structures are individually related to each other and form misleading profile.

4.4.7 Removal of the Stapes (Video 4.3)

The chorda tympani is dislocated downward (Fig. 4.5). Some stretching is applied to stick it to the tympanic membrane, laterally.

Measurement of the incus-footplate distance may not be necessary in experienced hands (Fig. 4.6). A gelfoam ball soaked by epinephrine

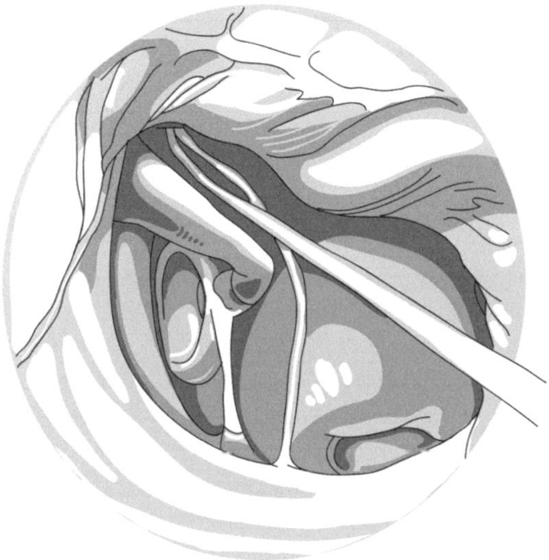

Fig. 4.5 Dislocation of the chorda tympani anteriorly and laterally

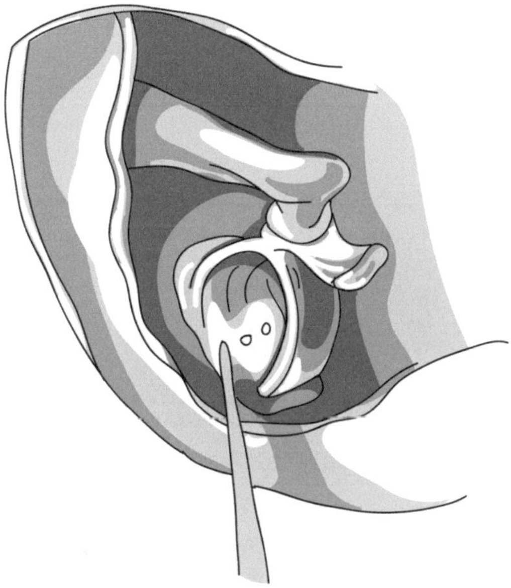

Fig. 4.7 Fenestration of the footplate

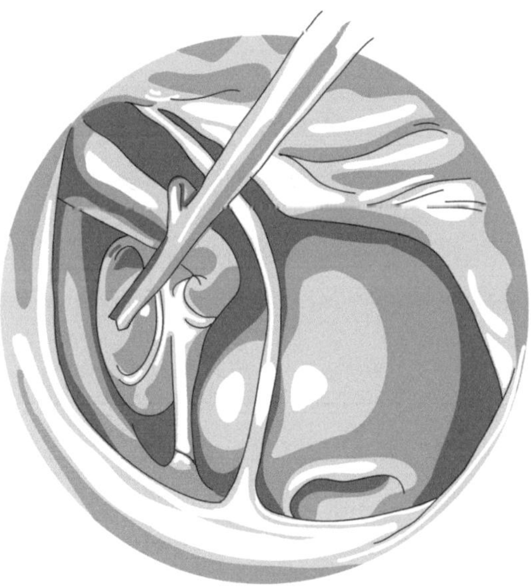

Fig. 4.6 Exact determination of the distance between the stapes footplate and the lenticular process of the incus by a measuring tool

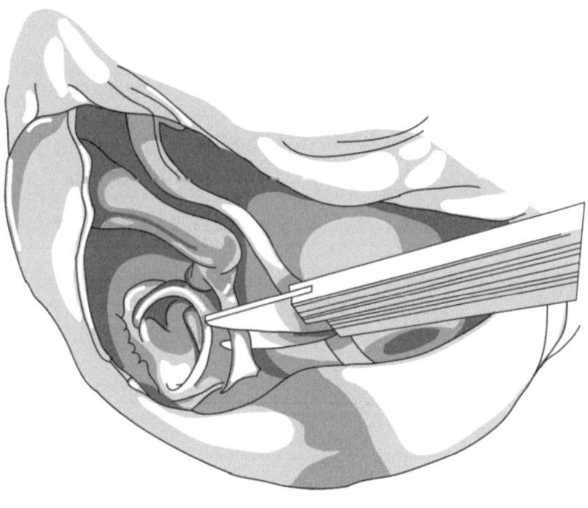

Fig. 4.8 Crossecting the tendon of the stapedius muscle

0.001 % solution is placed onto the footplate to avoid bleeding when elevating the mucosa which is highly vascularized and thickened in otosclerosis (Video 4.4). Fenestration of the footplate is preferably performed in the posterior one-third, right anterior to the posterior crus (Fig. 4.7, Video 4.5). It helps to clarify if gusher breaks out and makes possible to extract the footplate when the superstructure breaks down (Videos 4.6a, 4.6b, and 4.6c). An intense gusher makes stapedectomy impossible to execute, and the surgery should be continued as stapedotomy (Video 4.7). The incudostapedial joint is disarticulated by a needle, and the tendon of the stapedius muscle is cut (Fig. 4.8). Fine tilting movements of the stapes can be attempted anterior-to-posterior directions to try to mobilize the footplate. Sometimes this helps to extract the

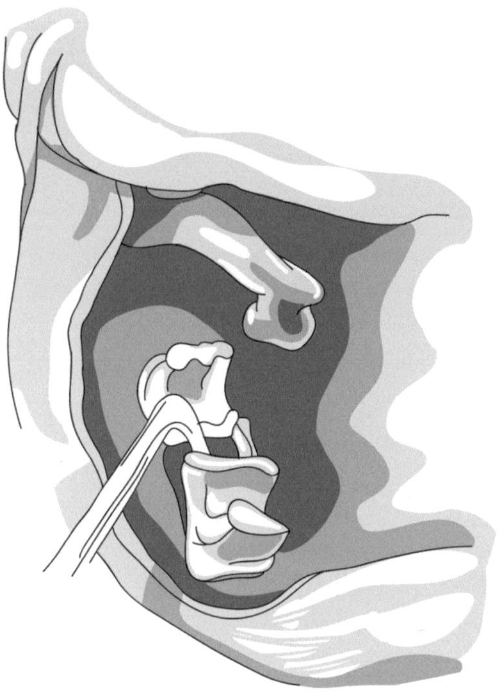

Fig. 4.9 Extraction of the stapes footplate

stapes in toto (Video 4.3). The superstructure, however, usually breaks down. It is pulled out by a hook. The footplate can be extracted by a footplate hook, sometimes in fragments (Fig. 4.9). Removal of a floating footplate can be attempted by a hook of 0.3 mm putting it in between the annular ligament and the footplate or piece of the footplate and extracting it that way or by a crocodile forceps (Video 4.6c). In otosclerosis the mucosa binds tightly to the footplate, and it usually doesn't allow footplate fragments to drop down into the vestibule. Non-otosclerotic stapes fixations may cause difficulties during stapedectomy. The adhesion between the mucosa and the footplate is loose, and the ankylosis between the oval window and the footplate is weak. This may lead to floating footplate that can be removed by drilling a hole in the promontory close to the niche, and by a hook the footplate can be removed. The surface tension of the perilymph in the vestibule also helps to prevent the footplate sunken into the vestibule.

4.4.8 Sealing the Oval Window (Video 4.8)

Some surgeons leave the oval window without coverage or they seal it by blood clot. This may lead to perilymph/CSF fistula because the clot is digested enzymatically on three to five postoperative days. Stapedectomy is total removal of the stapes footplate of a 3.75×1.75 mm surface. The hole should be covered. The options to harvest a graft are numerous. Fascia, perichondrium, compressed and dried connective tissue of any kind, and vein are equally used for sealing (Video 4.8). The graft should be thin because in case of revision surgery, the proper orientation may become difficult even with laser in hands. The connective tissue will be integrated to the bone and perhaps to the membranous labyrinth. Pulling the graft in the oval window can lead to damage of the labyrinth and to subsequent sensorineural hearing loss or deafness.

4.4.9 Placement of the Piston (Videos 4.9 and 4.10)

The piston length is between 4.5 and 5 mm. No measurement of the distance between the long process of the incus and the bottom of the oval window niche is necessary for an experienced surgeon. In case of a deep oval window niche, the length of the piston is 5 mm. The diameter is in the range of 0.4–0.8 mm. The depth of the piston immersion in the vestibule doesn't change the hearing outcome and is not responsible for less successful hearing restoration, postoperatively [36]. The Kurz Teflon-wire piston, I use, has 0.6 mm diameter in the interphase toward the vestibule (Video 4.10). Shea cup piston exists in 6×0.8 mm size. It is trimmed to 4.75 mm on an appropriate measuring table. As it is self-crimping, it adjusts the loop to the lenticular process without pressure (Video 4.9). The piston is placed into the operation field by the suction tube. The loop of the piston is taken posteriorly in a way that the axis of the piston and the suction tube gives an approximately 45° angle. Crimping the piston is the crucial step during the surgery.

The wire should be tight over the incus without breaking the long process down. First from posteriorly the wire is adjusted by the crimper to the incus. Second step is to finish circumferential tightening of the loop by moving the crimper downward from above. The mobility of the sound-transmitting system is checked by moving the handle of the malleus. The connection between the incus and the piston is also carefully controlled by the round window reflex. It should not be forgotten that around threshold sound intensity, the piston movement is in the nanometer range. Dropping the piston in the vestibule or pushing it too deep into the vestibule may result in sensorineural hearing loss and unsteadiness due to damage of the membranous labyrinth. Too short piston (<4.5 mm) may jump out from the oval window niche by intense pressure variations in the middle ear cavity especially when the niche is shallow. These can be prevented by careful manipulations in the oval window and choosing the appropriate length of the piston. Perilymph leak is rare but possible complication of stapedectomy. Closure of the opened vestibule by connective tissue after removal of the footplate effectively controls the potential leak. Breaking down the lenticular process of the piston requires reconstruction by ionomer cement or using angular piston. Alternatively, one may apply malleo-vestibulopexy by using long piston of 5.5–6 mm.

4.4.10 Repositioning the Chorda Tympani and the Tympanomeatal Flap

The chorda tympani is put on the piston wire hooked on the long process of the incus. It helps in vascular supply to the lenticular process. The auditory meatus is repositioned under otoscopic control. Any damage of the drum should be reconstructed by fascia and perichondrium graft. A silastic sheet is put on the tympanic membrane, and several gelfoam balls can be used to support the opening of the meatus. Antibiotic cream on gauze strip presses back the skinny meatus to the surrounding bone surfaces.

4.4.11 Skin Closure

Subcutaneous absorbable sutures are not necessary. The skin is closed by 3.0 prolene with interrupted knotted sutures.

4.5 Anatomical Disorders in the Operative Field

4.5.1 Dehiscent Facial Nerve Canal (Video 4.11)

The fallopian canal in its intratympanic course in the temporal bone runs horizontally first, above the oval window niche. Then underneath the lateral semicircular canal turns down to its vertical segment [26]. The bony facial nerve canal is covered in this segment by a thin bone covered by mucosal lining. Gross or microscopic dehiscences occur in a quite high frequency. Different studies by intraoperative observations or postmortem temporal bone dissections observed 1.8–70 % incidence of dehiscences in the fallopian canal in its horizontal course [3, 12, 16, 20, 32, 33]. Herniation of the nerve out of the canal may occur and may cause difficult surgical situation for making the hole on the stapes footplate and for placement of the piston as the nerve is unprotected by bony coverage. In the tympanic cavity, the highest incidence of the fallopian canal dehiscence was found around the oval window (horizontal segment) followed by the vertical segment [21]. It seems plausible in stapes fixation surgery that preoperative CT scanning of the temporal bone may help for the surgeon to be prepared for risky surgery when the nerve trunk partially or fully fills out the oval window niche. The value of the high-resolution CT scanning to image dehiscences in the fallopian canal, however, is limited [7]. When preoperatively the dehiscence can be imaged, a written consent is recommended from the patient as to call the attention to the risk of temporary facial weakness or possible facial paralysis. Overhanging facial nerve in the niche indicates a labyrinth fenestration nearby the oval window, downward to the middle segment of the stapes footplate by drilling. Dehiscent canal with the nerve in niveau of the bony canal may indicate angled piston wire to leave bigger room for the nerve. Facial palsy is a potential major complication of stapes surgery.

4.5.2 Obliterative Otosclerosis (Video 4.12)

In case of inactivated otosclerosis, the bone formation following the osteolytic active phase of the disease may lead to an unlimited bone production. The excessive bone formation fills out the oval window niche and may overgrow the rim of the niche. The stapes footplate cannot be identified, and the fallopian canal cannot be visualized also. Typically this bone is not very hard, but laser is not useful to make a hole on the promontory. The localization of the hole is best in the middle one-third of the footplate where the membranous labyrinth is far enough to avoid its damage [25]. The round window should be checked to exclude its ossification since the otosclerotic lesion may be so extended that it obliterates the round window. Using microdrill, the niche can be freed of bone keeping inferiorly on the promontory to avoid facial nerve trauma. Total stapedectomy is not recommended to perform as the large otosclerotic focus involves the membranous labyrinth and its removal can lead to profound sensorineural hearing loss.

4.5.3 Gusher (Video 4.7)

A mandatory episode in the order of steps of the surgical manipulation during stapedectomy is to make a hole in the stapes footplate before cutting the stapedius tendon and disarticulation of the incudostapedial joint. This is highly recommended even if preoperative CT scanning of the temporal bone was performed since the surgeon may not be certain whether malformations resulting in perilymph/CSF gusher may be expected intraoperatively [6]. Large vestibular aqueduct and osseous fistula in the internal auditory meatus (X chromosome-linked gusher) contraindicate stapedectomy. The excessive cerebrospinal fluid (CSF) leak excludes the closure of the oval window in a way which results in hearing restoration. The CSF leak coming out the oval window under pressure takes away the fascia for coverage. An oversized piece of muscle or fat should be plugged into the window, and fibrin glue is used to fix it. It results in conductive hearing loss that may exceed the preoperative air-bone gap. Making a hole in the footplate only will show that a gusher is present, and under continuous suction, we can place a fascia upon it, and the piston can plug the hole (Video 4.7). The leak can be controlled and the hearing is restored.

4.5.4 High Jugular Bulb (Fig. 4.10)

A high jugular bulb is distinguished from an asymmetrically large jugular bulb by its roof reaching above the internal auditory meatus. A run of the high-riding jugular bulb has an intact sigmoid plate – a thin plate of bone separating the jugular bulb from the middle ear cavity. This can only be appreciated on thin slice bone algorithm CT and is too thin to appreciate on MRI. If the

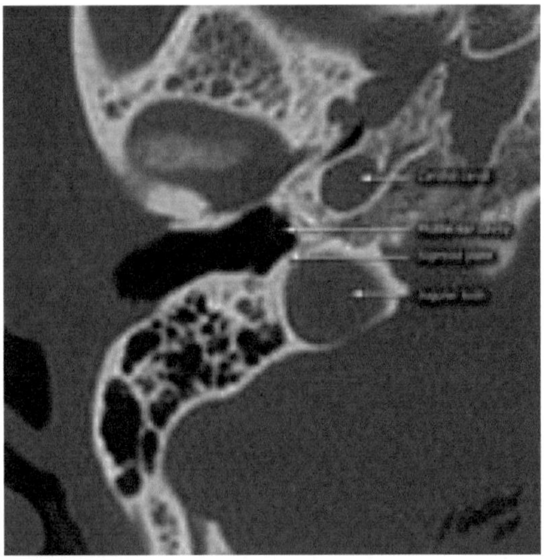

Fig. 4.10 High jugular bulb in an axial CT: *white arrows* show the bulb, the bone plate separating the bulb from the middle ear cavity, the middle ear, and the internal carotid artery (from *downward* to *upward*) (From www.Radiopaedia.org)

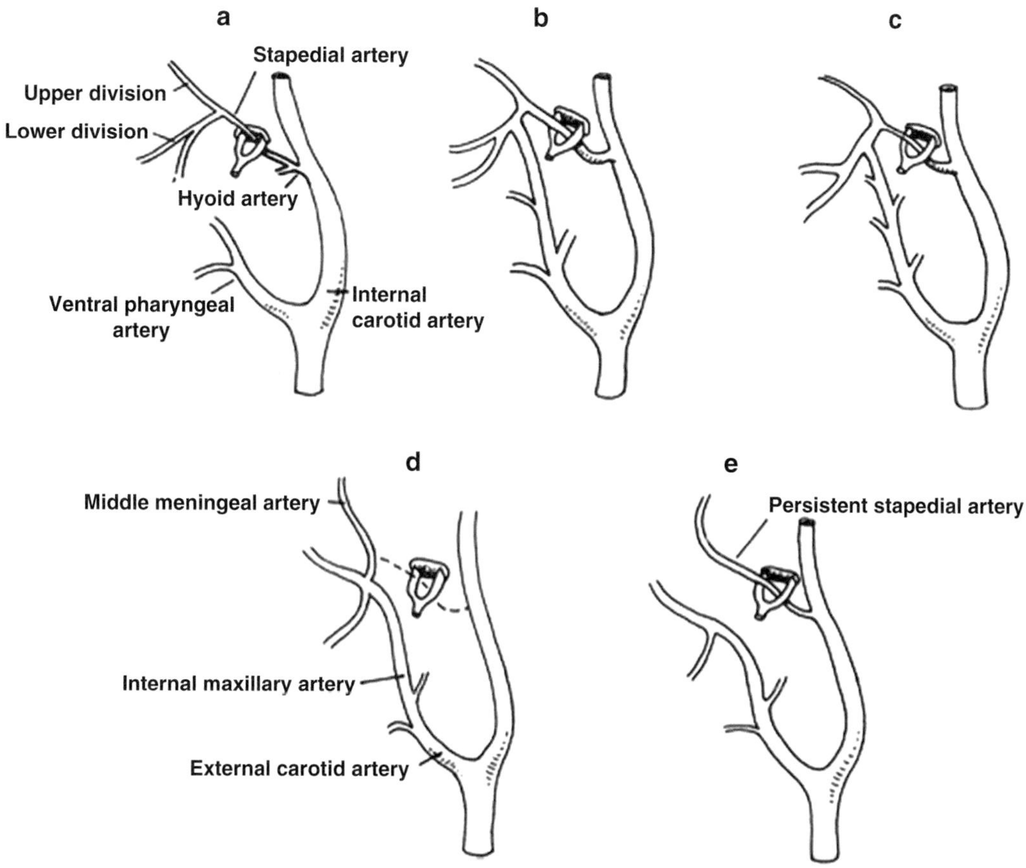

Fig. 4.11 Different variations of the stapedial artery as it derives from the internal carotid artery and runs between the crura of the stapes toward different branches of the external carotid artery [29]

sigmoid plate is deficient, the bulb is free to protrude into the middle ear cavity. This can exclude the surgical intervention in the oval window niche area.

4.5.5 Persistent Stapedial Artery (Fig. 4.11)

The persistent stapedial artery is a rare anomaly. It traverses the oval window niche right above the stapes footplate between the crura [29]. Coagulation of the artery is contraindicated because it leads to profuse bleeding. The artery may leave sufficient place for making a hole on the posterior segment of the footplate; otherwise, it is best to finish the surgery at this point and providing hearing rehabilitation by hearing aid. Sometimes only the obliterated remnant of the artery is found [18].

4.6 Partial Stapedectomy

It provides the same hearing gain as total stapedectomy in all frequencies except 4 kHz where partial stapedectomy is better [22]. The surgical steps are similar to those described in stapedectomy. Usually the otosclerotic focus in otosclerotic stapes fixations develops in the anterior pole of the stapes footplate. Consequently, a partial removal of the footplate is removal of the posterior half of the footplate. This is easy to execute, easier than a total removal. In otosclerosis, the risk of a floating footplate remnant is low because of the tight adhesion in the anterior pole of the footplate. Non-otosclerotic stapes fixations should be managed differently. In these cases no morphological integration between the footplate and the oval window develops through the annular ligament. The non-otosclerotic fixation process (e.g., calcification) results in a footplate bulky. The interface between the footplate and the oval window is smooth. Partial stapedectomy in these non-otosclerotic fixation cases will reduce the stiffness between the facing bone surfaces letting the anterior half of the footplate mobile. It risks the footplate dropping down into the vestibule. Non-otosclerotic stapes fixations are also characterized by a thin, nonvascularized, mucosal lining in the oval window niche. That doesn't help to keep up the footplate from dislocating.

4.7 Alternative Stapedectomy Techniques

4.7.1 Stapedectomy with Preservation of the Stapedius Muscle Tendon

A conventional stapedectomy during this type of surgery will not extend to removal or crosscutting the tendon of the stapedius muscle. The muscle is inserted into the head of the stapes. Physiologically its contraction pulls the head of the stapes backward resulting in an elevation of the anterior half of the footplate with simultaneous depression of the posterior half into the vestibule. The ossicular chain becomes more rigid which attenuates the magnitude of the sound transmission up to 2700 Hz. Preserving the muscle during stapedectomy may exhibit some tension application to the ossicular chain which is, however, limited as the articulation between the head of the stapes and the lenticular process of the incus allows some mobility. The effective length change of the muscle during contraction will not exceed more than fragments of a mm. Conversely, preservation of the tendon results in a gross 15 dB loudness discomfort level increase [9], only.

4.7.2 Posterior Crus Stapedectomy

This procedure saves the stapedial crura, or at least the posterior crus, in its full length. The crus is carefully transected right at the level of the footplate. The footplate is removed. The opened vestibule is covered by the conventional way with fascia, vein, or other type of connective tissue. Instead of inserting a piston, the posterior stapes crus is applied as an interpositum between the incus and the vestibule. Although good hearing results were reported [34], the procedure can easily result in a short interpositum effect which produces air-bone gap along time.

4.8 Postoperative Care

Stapes surgery without complication (perilymph fistula, facial palsy, vertigo) is a daycare procedure. The external auditory meatus is filled with antibacterial cream soaked gauze strip, and the tympanic membrane is covered by a silastic sheet. The gauze strip is removed along with suture removal at the seventh day, in endaural approach. The silastic and some gelfoam balls upon it are removed 3 weeks after surgery. Audiometric control of hearing restoration success can be attempted on the operating table, already. This will exhibit a very approximate improvement level but is convincing for no hearing loss due to surgery.

4.9 Advantages and Disadvantages of Stapedectomy Over Stapedotomy

Advantages of stapedectomy:

- Good hearing results at the speech frequencies and negligible hearing loss at high frequencies (4–8 kHz)
- Footplate sample for histological diagnosis (identification of the disease)
- Footplate sample for research as to pathomechanism and prevention

- Tinnitus suppression
- Removal of the stapedial part of the otosclerotic focus and decreasing the release of inflammatory mediators into the inner ear

Disadvantages of stapedectomy:

- Poorer high-frequency hearing
- Higher risk of vertigo

Advantages of stapedotomy:

- Good hearing results in all frequencies
- No vertigo
- Tinnitus suppression
- Less risk for floating footplate

Disadvantages of stapedotomy:

- No histological diagnosis
- Sensorineural hearing loss on a long run since the whole focus remains in place

References

1. Arnold A, Fawzy T, Steinhoff HJ, Kiefer J, Arnold W. Influence of a totally open oval window on bone conduction in otosclerosis. Audiol Neuro Otol. 2011;16:23–8.
2. Bauer M, Pytel J, Vona I, Gerlinger I. Long term results of the use of autogenous cortical bone columella to replace the stapes at stapedectomy. Eur Arch Otorhinolaryngol. 2011;268:671–5.
3. Baxter A. Dehiscence of the fallopian canal. J Laryngol. 1971;85:524–7.
4. Carhart R, Hayes C. Clinical reliability of bone conduction audiometry. Laryngoscope. 1949;59:1084–101.
5. Coker NJ, Ator GA, Jenkins HA, Neblett CR. Carbon dioxide laser stapedotomy:a histopathologic study. Am J Otolaryngol. 1986;7:253–7.
6. Crouchy L, Callonnec F, Bouchetemblé P, Tollard E, Dehesdin D, Marie JP. Preoperative computed tomography scan may fail to predict perilymphatic gusher. Ann Otol Rhinol Laryngol. 2013;122:374–7.
7. Di Martino E, Sellhaus B, Haenser J, Schlegel JG, Westhofen M, Prescher A. Fallopian canal dehiscences: a survey of clinical anatomical findings. Eur Arch Otorhinolaryngol. 2005;262:120–6.
8. Glasscock ME, Storper IS, Haynes DS, Bohrer PS. Stapedectomy in profound cochlear loss. Laryngoscope. 1996;106:831–3.
9. Gros A, Zargi M, Vatovec J. Does it make sense to preserve the stapedius muscle during surgical treatment for otosclerosis? J Laryngol Otol. 2000;114: 930–4.
10. Hall A, Rytzner C. Stapedectomy and autotransplantation of ossicles. Acta Otolaryngol. 1957;47: 318–24.
11. Hausler R, Messerli A, Romano V, Burkhalter R, Weber HP, Altermatt HJ. Experimental and clinical results of fiberoptic argon laser stapedotomy. Eur Arch Otorhinolaryngol. 1996;253:193–200.
12. Hough J. Congenital malformations of the middle ear. Arch Otolaryngol. 1963;78:335–43.
13. House WJ, Cunningham DC. Otosclerosis. In: Cumming CW, Flint PW, Harker LA, Haughey BH, Richardson MA, Robbins KT, et al., editors. Cummings otolaryngology head and neck surgery. 5th ed. Philadelphia: Elsevier Mosby; 2010. p. 1887–2035.
14. Jovanovic S, Anft D, Schonfeld U, Berghaus A, Scherer H. Influence of CO2 laser application to the guinea-pig cochlea on compound action potentials. Am J Otol. 1999;20:166–73.
15. Jovanovic S, Schonfeld U, Fischer R, et al. Thermic effects in the "vestibule" during laser stapedotomy with pulsed laser systems. Lasers Surg Med. 1998;23: 7–17.
16. Kaplan J. Congenital dehiscences of the fallopian canal in middle ear surgery. Arch Otolaryngol. 1960;72:197–200.
17. Karosi T, Kónya J, Z Szabó L, Sziklai I. Anti-measles immunoglobulin G for serologic diagnosis of otosclerotic hearing loss. Laryngoscope. 2006;118:488–93.
18. Karosi T, Szabó LZ, Petkó M, Sziklai I. Otosclerotic stapes with three crura and persisting stapedial artery. Otol Neurotol. 2008;29:1043–4.
19. Massey BL, Kennedy RJ, CShelton C. Stapedectomy outcomes: titanium versus teflon wire prosthesis. Laryngoscope. 2005;115:249–52.
20. Moreano EH, Paparelly MM, Zelterman D, Goicoolea MV. Prevalence of facial canal dehiscence and of persistent stapedial artery in the human middle ear: a report of 1000 temporal bones. Laryngoscope. 1994;104:309–20.
21. Perez B, Campos ME, Rivero J, Campos DL, Lopez-Aguado D. Incidence of dehiscences in the fallopian canal. Int J Pediatr Otorhinolaryngol. 1997;40:51–60.
22. Persson P, Harder H, Magnusson B. Hearing results in otosclerosis surgery after partial stapedectomy, total stapedectomy and stapedotomy. Acta Otolaryngol. 1997;117:94–9.
23. Rizer FM, Lippy WH. Evolution of techniques on stapedectomy from the total stapedectomy to the small fenestra stapedotomy. Otolaryngol Clin N Am. 1993;26:443–51.
24. Rosen S, Bergman M. The first one hundred cases of hearing improvement after stapes mobilization – a long term report. Laryngoscope. 1959;69:1960–5.
25. Saunders NC, Fagan PA. Promontory drilling in stapedectomy: an anatomical study. Otol Neurotol. 2006;27:776–80.

26. Schuknecht HF. Pathology of the ear. Cambridge: Harvard University Press; 1974. p. 192–5.
27. Schuknecht HF. Stapedectomy. Boston: Little Brown; 1971.
28. Shea Jr JJ. Fenestration of the oval window. Ann Otol Rhinol Laryngol. 1958;67:932–51.
29. Silbergleit R, Quint DJ, Mehta BA, Patel SC, Metes JJ, Noujaim SE. The persistent stapedial artery. Artery Am J Neuroradiol. 2000;21:572–7.
30. Slattery WH, House JW. Prostheses for stapes surgery. Otolaryngol Clin N Am. 1995;28:253–64.
31. St Martin MB, Rubinstein EM, Hirsch BE. High frequency sensorineural hearing loss after stapedectomy. Otol Neurotol. 2008;29:447–52.
32. Takahashi H, Sando I. Facial canal dehiscence: histologic study and computer reconstruction. Ann Otol Rhinol Laryngol. 1992;101:925–30.
33. Tange RA, de Bruijn AJG. Dehiscences of the horizontal segment of the facial ca in otosclerosis. ORL. 1997;59:277–9.
34. Vartiainen E, Nuutinen J, Karjalainen S, Pellinen P. Posterior crus stapedectomy. J Laryngol Otol. 1993;107:795–7.
35. Wegner I, Kamalski DMA, Tange RA, Vincent R, Stegeman I, van der Heijden GJM, Grolman WD. Laser versus conventional fenestration in stapedotomy for otosclerosis: a systematic review. Laryngoscope. 2014;124:1687–93.
36. Yehudai N, Masoud S, Most T, Luntz M. Depth of stapes prosthesis in the vestibule: baseline values and correlation with stapedectomy outcome. Acta Otolaryngol. 2010;130:904–8.

5 Laser Stapedotomy

S. Jovanovic and A.E. Albers

5.1 Introduction

Otosclerosis is characterized by an abnormal growing and remodeling of the bony labyrinth capsule and may occur on one side or bilaterally. The pathologic remodeling of enchondral bone manifests most frequently in the anterior part of the oval window niche. A complete bonification of the oval window has been termed obliterative otosclerosis. The rare incidence of malignant otosclerosis is defined by bony remodeling and areas of bonification in the area of the round and oval window and the temporal bone.

The etiology of otosclerosis has still not been completely resolved, and there are probably multiple causes including genetic, metabolic, and endocrinologic factors and viral infection or postinfectious immunologic reactions.

Clinically, otosclerosis manifests by a slowly progressing air-bone gap that may be combined with sensorineural hearing loss. The latter is typically most prominent at 2 kHz (Carhart notch) and is possibly due to a decreased resonance of middle ear structures [31]. In 10 % of cases, an isolated sensorineural hearing loss is observed that has been termed cochlear otosclerosis. The air-bone gap can reach up to 40 dB HL and is more prominent in the low-frequency range. In about half of the patients, tinnitus and sometimes vertigo are present [5, 29]. A typical constellation of symptoms is an air-bone gap with sensorineural hearing loss at 2 kHz, a normal ear microscopy finding combined with an absent stapedius reflex on the affected side.

A successful treatment of otosclerosis by stapedotomy and reconstruction of the ossicle chain is characterized by a closure of the air-bone gap, improvement of sensorineural hearing loss, and frequently reduction of tinnitus.

5.1.1 Role of Different Laser Systems for Stapedotomy

A perforation of the stapes footplate with a diameter of 0.5–0.7 mm is necessary to place a prosthesis into the vestibulum. The diameter of an Argon or KTP laser beam is 0.15 mm. Therefore, several small perforations have to be placed adjacent to each other to achieve the desired diameter (Fig. 5.2, left). Overlapping laser applications should be avoided since the laser irradiation is not absorbed by the perilymph. Residual bone (e.g., bony bridges) can be removed with instruments.

S. Jovanovic, MD, PhD (✉)
Krankenhaus Bethel Berlin, Promenadenstr.3-5, Berlin 12207, Germany
e-mail: sergije.jovanovic@gmx.de

A.E. Albers, MD, PhD
Hals-Nasen-Ohrenklinik, Charité Campus Benjamin Franklin, Hindenburgdamm 30, Berlin 12200, Germany
e-mail: andreas.albers@charite.de

I. Sziklai (ed.), *Surgery of Stapes Fixations*, DOI 10.1007/978-3-319-28576-4_5

The CO_2 laser has a beam diameter of 0.18 mm, and since the irradiation is absorbed by perilymph [17], overlapping applications with a multishot technique are possible and result in a rounded shape of the perforation (Fig. 5.2, middle). However, irradiation of an empty vestibule (e.g., after accidental suction of the perilymph) poses the risk of inner-ear damage and should be avoided [17].

The development of laser-scanning devices that are combined with a CO_2 laser has led to the development of the one-shot laser stapedotomy. Ideally, this technique allows to perforate the stapes footplate with a single-laser application. The scanner guides the focused beam over the area to be perforated. The application of this technique results in a round perforation and minimizes the risk of thermal and acoustic damage [12, 16].

In the following, this technique will be explained for primary and revision stapedotomy.

5.1.2 One-Shot CO_2-Laser Stapedotomy

5.1.2.1 CO_2 Laser

In continuous wave (cw) mode, the CO_2 laser is effective for removing soft tissue, and it can vaporize thin bony structures when focused to a small spot [16]. One advantage of the CO_2 laser is its strong absorption by water, resulting in a penetration depth of only 0.01 mm from the irradiated surface. This property of CO_2-laser light is particularly useful in stapes surgery since the perilymph completely absorbs the CO_2-laser energy and thus protects the inner ear structures from direct injury.

5.1.2.2 Micromanipulator

The CO_2-laser light is delivered to the operative site through an articulated arm and a micromanipulator (AcuSpot™ 712 micromanipulator, Lumenis Ltd., Yokneam, Israel) coupled to an operating microscope. A joystick attached to the micromanipulator is used to move the laser beam within the operative field.

The CO_2 laser can be used with micromanipulators allowing a spot size of 0.18–0.2 mm at a working distance of 250 mm. With a good beam profile and perfect alignment of the helium neon (HeNe) aiming beam with the CO_2 treatment beam, precise microsurgical work can be carried out on middle ear structures.

5.1.2.3 Scanner System

When a CO_2-laser beam is directed by microprocessor-controlled rotating mirrors known as scanner systems (SurgiTouch, Lumenis Ltd., Yokneam, Israel), the beam is automatically tracked in a spiral-shaped pattern within a designated pulse duration. In this way, the CO_2 laser can deliver high power densities evenly over a relatively large treatment area with minimal collateral effects. At a working distance of 250 or 275 mm, the size of the treated area can be freely selected in accordance with the local anatomic configuration and the desired size of the perforation.

5.1.2.4 Laser Settings

For the surgery, a CO_2 laser (type 40c, Lumenis Ltd., Yokneam, Israel) equipped with a scanner and a micromanipulator is used. Effective and safe laser parameters are available for the requirements of primary stapedotomy and revision cases (Table 5.1), where the vaporization of bone and soft tissue formations is also necessary [17, 24]. For all surgeries, the laser is used in continuous wave mode at a working distance of 250 mm with a focused beam diameter of 180 μm. Since the transmission of CO_2-laser irradiation via the hinged mirror arm and micromanipulator involves power losses varying from 20 to 30 % depending on the system used, the power indicated on the laser is higher than the effective power that is actually applied to the tissue. The data specified in Table 5.1 correspond to the powers applied to the target tissue.

5.2 One-Shot CO_2-Laser Stapedotomy

The one-shot CO_2-laser stapedotomy is possible in general or local anesthesia combined with sedation of the patient. While it is generally accepted that general anesthesia is advantageous

Table 5.1 Effective laser energy parameters for revision stapes surgery [24] (specified powers correspond to real powers at the end of the application system)

Anatomic structure	Effective power [W]	Power density [W/cm²]	Pulse duration [s]	Power mode	Beam diameter [mm]	Number of pulses	Perforation diameter [mm]
Parameters for one-shot CO_2-laser stapedotomy							
Stapes tendon	2	8000	0.05	cw	0.18	2–3	
Incudostapedial joint	6	24,000	0.05	cw	0.18	8–14	
Anterior/posterior crus of the stapes	6	24,000	0.05	cw	0.18	4–8	
Stapes footplate	20–22[a]	80,000–88,000	0.03–0.05	cw	0.5; 0.6, 0.7	1	0.5–0.7
Parameters for revision one-shot CO_2-laser stapedotomy							
Soft tissue	1–2	4000–8000	0.05	cw	0.18		
Connective tissue neo-membrane	1–2 (multiple single shots)	4000–8000	0.05	cw	0.18	6–12	0.5–0.7
	or	or	or		or	or	
	4–8[a] ("one-shot technique")	16,000–32,000	0.03–0.05		0.5, 0.6 or 0.7	1	
Bony stapes footplate	6	24,000	0.05	cw	0.18	1	0.5–0.7
	or	or	or		or		
	20–22[a] ("one-shot technique")	80,000–88,000	0.03–0.05		0.5, 0.6 or 0.7		

[a]For the one-shot technique, the SurgiTouch™-Scanner was used

if patients are incompliant, some surgeons argue that local anesthesia has the advantage of intraoperative hearing tests. Due to the highly reproducible hearing improvement and low incidence of complications in our view, the latter can be neglected. Eventually, preferences of the surgeon and patient and last but not least economic considerations may play a role.

5.2.1 One-Shot Laser Stapedotomy in Primary Cases

5.2.1.1 Exposure of Middle Ear Structures

The external auditory canal is infiltrated with 1 % lidocaine (Xylocaine) with 1:200,000 epinephrine, and the tympanomeatal flap is elevated to gain access to the middle ear. The canal bone covering the oval window niche is removed with a sharp House curette or diamond bur, preserving the chorda tympani. Sufficient access to the oval window is gained when the pyramidal process and tympanic segment of the facial nerve are clearly visible. Before the CO_2 laser is used, alignment of the HeNe-laser aiming beam and the invisible CO_2-laser beam is probed by test shots on a wooden spatula (Fig. 5.1a).

As described in the following, the stapedial tendon, incudostapedial joint, and crura are vaporized, and the footplate is perforated with the CO_2-laser beam by using the noncontact technique.

5.2.1.2 Removal of the Stapes Superstructure

Stapedial tendon The stapedial tendon is vaporized with two or three separate pulses of 0.05 s duration at 2 W (power density 8000 W/cm²) (Fig. 5.1b) [1]. In some cases, it may be possible to preserve the tendon if anatomic conditions are favorable.

Incudostapedial joint The incudostapedial joint is generally separated by conventional means in cases with complete stapes fixation. If

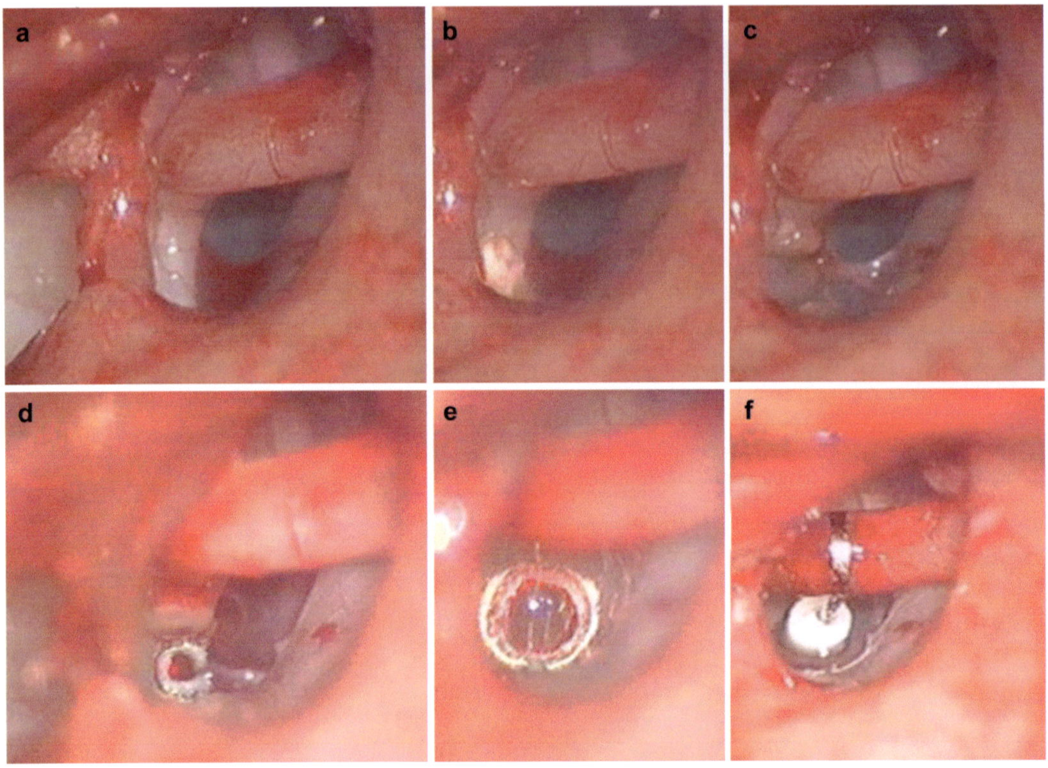

Fig. 5.1 (**a**) Middle ear cavity after exposure of the stapes. (**b**) Cutting of the stapes tendon. (**c**) Incudostapedial joint after separation. (**d**) Transection of the posterior crus. (**e**) Perforated stapes footplate. (**f**) Placed prosthesis

the footplate is only partially fixed, laser-assisted separation of the joint is performed. The joint is opened with 8–14 pulses of 0.05 s duration at 6 W (power density 24,000 W/cm^2), vaporizing the stapes capitulum [2]. Since the CO_2-laser beam often does not strike the joint precisely at a perpendicular angle, the joint should also be probed with a manual instrument, to separate remaining connections between the lenticular process and stapes capitulum (Fig. 5.1c) [3].

Posterior crus The bone of the posterior crus is generally thicker, longer, and more curved than the anterior crus. It is transected close to the footplate with four to eight pulses of 0.05 s duration at 6 W (power density 24,000 W/cm^2). During the separation of the incudostapedial joint and the transection of the posterior crus, care should be taken that the laser beam does not accidentally strike middle ear structures lying in the path of the beam (e.g., footplate, canal of the facial nerve). This can be prevented by filling the middle ear with physiologic saline solution or by covering these structures with a moist gelatin sponge (Gelita or Spongostan). If the posterior crus remnant is still too long after the suprastructure has been removed, it can be vaporized to the level of the footplate using the same laser parameters to obtain better posterior exposure of the footplate (Fig. 5.1d).

Anterior crus The anterior crus of the stapes is fractured with a small hook. If the complete or a part of the anterior crus is visible, it is vaporized with the CO_2 laser using the same parameters as for the posterior crus. If this does not completely transect the crus, the vaporized site can be fractured using controlled pressure on the small hook. This virtually eliminates the danger of mobilizing the footplate or even partially or completely extracting it. The stapes superstructure is then removed with a small forceps. Again, it is

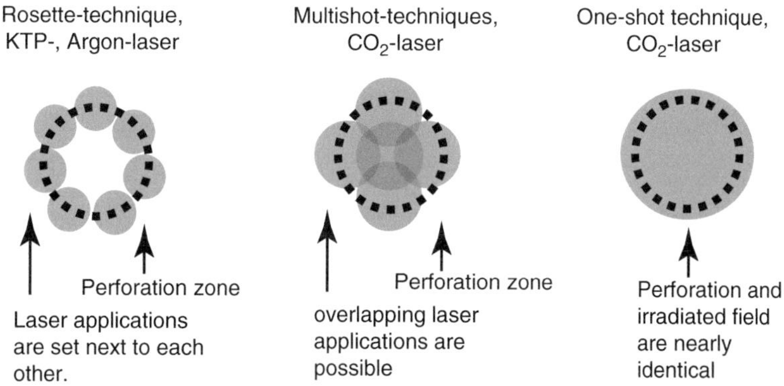

Fig. 5.2 Overview of the application pattern of different lasers (KTP, Argon laser (*left*), CO_2-laser multishot technique (*middle*), and CO_2-laser one-shot technique (*right*))

advisable to protect the surrounding structures (footplate, canal of the facial nerve) as described above.

5.2.1.3 Stapedotomy

After the suprastructure has been removed, the stapedotomy opening is created in the posterior half of the footplate. The goal is to create a round perforation of 0.5–0.7 mm in diameter, applying the beam either in a single application (one-shot technique) or in a slightly overlapping pattern (multishot technique).

It is possible to create a smooth, round perforation of 0.5–0.7 mm in diameter in approximately more than 70 % of cases with a single 20–22-W laser application of 0.03–0.05-s duration [17]. In cases where a single application does not create the desired perforation diameter, a second shot can safely be applied to the same site with the scanner. Alternatively multiple shots can be applied without a scanner (Fig. 5.2, middle).

If a scanner is not available, the footplate can be perforated using a multishot technique. For this, the CO_2-laser beam is set to 180 μm in diameter, and a power of 6 W and pulse duration of 0.05 s is used. Depending on the thickness of the footplate, 6–12 shots are needed to create an adequate perforation.

Care should be taken that the vestibule is filled with perilymph to ensure adequate protection for inner ear structures and to prevent damage from direct irradiation. If the perilymph is inadvertently suctioned from the vestibule, no additional laser energy should be applied to the footplate. Before further laser treatment, it may become necessary to fill the vestibule with physiologic saline solution.

5.2.1.4 Placement of the Prosthesis

A prosthesis of 0.4–0.6 mm in diameter and a length of 4.25–4.75 mm is inserted into the perforation and connected to the long process of the incus. Depending on the type of the prosthesis, different techniques are used (Table 5.2). The diameter of the prosthesis should be 0.1–0.2 mm smaller than the perforation.

Next, the oval window niche is sealed with connective tissue or clotted blood [27], and finally the tympanic membrane and the tympanomeatal flap are replaced, and, silicone strips, an antibiotic-containing packing, is placed and the wound is closed.

5.2.1.5 Choice of the Prosthesis

The length of the replaced prosthesis is determined by measuring the distance from the lower surface of the incus to the vestibule and by adding 0.2 mm. The most commonly used size is 4.5–4.75 mm. The length of the prosthesis is chosen to extend 0.1–0.2 mm into the perforation to prevent migration. Table 5.2 provides an overview of popular prostheses.

5.2.1.6 Postoperative Care

All packings and stitches can be removed 8–10 days after the operation. A pure-tone hearing test is performed on all patients 1 day prior the operation. To assess the inner ear function, a hearing test should be performed 1 day after the

Table 5.2 Material and fixation method of popular stapes prostheses

Prosthesis (company)	Material	Fixation
K-Piston (Kurz)	Titan	Fixation with McGee forceps
Platin-Teflon piston (Spiggle & Theiss)	Platin and Teflon	Fixation with McGee forceps
Platin-prostheses type "House" (Spiggle & Theiss)	Platin	Fixation with McGee forceps
CliP® Piston àWengen titan stapes prosthesis (Kurz)	Titan	Self-fixating
Nitinol piston (band-shape) (audio technology)	Nitinol	Self-fixating
NiTiBOND® stapes prosthesis (Kurz)	Nitinol	Fixation through heat induced bending and clipping
Nitinol prostheses (Gyrus ACMI ENT)	Nitinol wire and Teflon shaft	Heating of the prosthesis to <45 °C[a]
Super elastic Nitinol-Teflon prosthesis (Spiggle & Theiss)	Nitinol and Teflon	Heating of the prosthesis to <45 °C[a]

[a]Laser: 3 × 1 W, cutting mode 0.05 s pulse duration

operation and repeatedly during the first postoperative year. Air conduction should be assessed approximately 6 weeks after the operation. A continuous improvement of the air conduction can be expected during the first postoperative year.

5.2.2 Solutions for Difficult Anatomic Constellations

5.2.2.1 Obliterative Otosclerosis

The incidence of obliterative otosclerosis is between 2 and 10 % of all cases [10, 25]. Drilling through a thick footplate obliterating the oval window niche can cause vibration-induced inner ear trauma. With the CO_2 laser, on the other hand, it is possible to perforate a stapes footplate, regardless of its thickness or degree of fixation, without mechanical trauma to the inner ear.

The settings are the same as used for a laser stapedotomy. After the suprastructure has been removed, the otosclerotic foci obliterating the oval window niche are uniformly removed by several laser applications with the scanner. This procedure is continued until the lateral margins of the oval window can be clearly identified [7]. Lower laser powers may have to be used in the periphery of the window niche to avoid accidentally entering the inner ear. Large amounts of char are produced as the bony material is vaporized. Since crystalline char reflects the CO_2-laser light reducing its ablative effect, it should be removed with a suitable instrument. The vestibule in the posterior part of the oval window niche is opened with one or several laser applications [7] using the same parameters as for a one-shot stapedotomy. If the diameter of the perforation is too small to accommodate the prosthesis, the opening can be enlarged either by re-treating the same site with the scanner or by applying a concentric pattern of laser applications without the scanner.

5.2.2.2 Overhanging Facial Nerve

An overhanging tympanic facial nerve segment, whether covered by bone or occasionally exposed, can be a serious obstacle to surgical access. If the facial nerve is covered by bone, the CO_2 laser can be carefully applied tangentially at low powers (1–2 W), using pulse durations of 0.05 s to remove the bone. Scanner settings of 4–5 W, 0.03–0.04 s pulse duration, and 0.3–0.4 mm scanner diameter are safe and effective. Occasionally, this treatment is already sufficient to obtain the necessary access to the footplate. Complete removal of bony covering should be avoided to protect the nerve from accidental laser irradiation and to prevent a prolapse of the nerve through a defect, decreasing vision of the footplate even more.

In cases where the facial canal completely obstructs access to the oval window niche and removal of the frequently very thin bone will not significantly improve access, or if the tympanic facial nerve segment is not covered by bone at all, use of the laser should be suspended in favor of, e.g., a conventional stapedotomy with a curved perforator. Another option for difficult access is to redirect the CO_2-laser beam with a mirror. This may enable the surgeon to perforate a footplate that is not directly accessible to the laser.

5.2.2.3 Overhanging Promontory

Narrowing of the oval window niche by an overhanging promontory wall projecting into the niche generally poses only a minor surgical problem. Using the precautionary measures described earlier (covering the footplate with saline solution or moist gelatin sponge), the bone can be ablated with a tangentially directed laser beam using the parameters given above to provide a direct view of the oval window niche.

During removal of the overhanging promontory bone, care should be taken to avoid opening the scala tympani. The risk of opening the scalar tympani and damaging the inner ear with the CO_2-laser beam is lower (absorption of the laser energy by the perilymph and a low penetration depth of 0.01 mm) than if, e.g., a diamond bur is used.

5.2.2.4 Inaccessible Footplate

If the footplate is not accessible, for example, due to an abnormal course of the facial nerve or a vascular anomaly, restoration of the sound conduction chain may require fenestration of the promontory using a technique described by Plester et al. Apart from using the CO_2 laser to create the perforation, the surgery is done according to conventional technique. However, the authors have no personal experience with CO_2-laser perforation of the promontory, since so far access to the oval window niche was gained in all cases.

5.2.2.5 Floating Footplate

In the course of a conventional stapedotomy, it may happen that the footplate is mobilized. In this case, the creation of an adequate perforation with conventional means might prove difficult. One solution is to perform a stapedectomy. The other, more preferable option is to perforate the footplate using the CO_2 laser as described above [21].

5.2.3 One-Shot Laser Stapedotomy in Revision Cases

To restore hearing in revision stapedotomy, a precise identification and correction of the underlying abnormality without impairment of the inner ear function is necessary. A number of reasons alone or in combination can cause the conductive hearing loss after primary stapedotomy: a displaced, fixed, or loose prosthesis; a subluxated, fixed, or eroded malleus or incus; and fibrosis or regrowth of otosclerotic bone in the oval window niche [4, 28]. For an accurate diagnosis, it is necessary to visualize the malleus and incus and to clear the oval window niche from connective tissue until the margins of the footplate are visible. Finally, the position of the piston in the stapedotomy opening has to be checked.

Since the introduction of otologic lasers in stapes surgery, success rates of stapes-revision surgery have greatly improved. Postoperative hearing results have become nearly comparable to those obtained after primary stapedotomy, and the rate of postoperative complications is greatly reduced. This may be due to the enhanced ability of the revising surgeon to safely identify and treat the causes for conductive hearing loss was less than even after multiple revisions. The risk of profound postoperative sensorineural hearing loss in several large series of laser revision cases is less than 1 % independent of the laser system used [4, 6, 8, 9, 18, 20, 22, 23, 32]. While in conventional stapes surgery a closure of the air-bone gap of 20 dB or less is achieved in 49–85 %, the use of lasers improved the outcome to 70–92 % [26]. From these data, an early revision can be encouraged to prevent incus erosion caused by a dislocated prosthesis. In these cases, the incus continues to vibrate against the fixed prosthesis causing the erosion. In cases of a perilymph fistula, a delay of closure will increase the risk of sensorineural hearing loss, since the fistula will not close spontaneously [19].

In contrast to primary stapes surgery, in revision surgery not only bone has to be vaporized but also soft tissue filling the middle ear cavity including the oval niche. Therefore, a laser with physical properties suited for vaporization of bone and soft tissue should be used. A CO_2 laser meets these requirements. During vaporization of connective tissue in the oval niche or direct irradiation of the prosthesis, heat may be directly conducted to the vestibulum if the piston is still in the stapedotomy opening. Therefore, excessive direct irradiation should be avoided. In previous studies, we and others have experimentally shown that the CO_2 laser can be used safely and effectively [11–17, 30].

However, to further reduce the risk of damage, the authors advise a surgical technique that minimizes mechanical manipulation of the conductive chain and consequently reduces trauma and heat conduction to the inner ear structures.

5.3 Surgical Technique of Revision Laser Stapedotomy

5.3.1 Exposure of Middle Ear Structures

The tympanomeatal flap is elevated as described in Sect. 2.1.1 and the middle ear structures are inspected. In some instances, for proper exposure of the posterior half of the oval niche, the posterior wall of the outer ear canal has to be further reduced, and the chorda tympani requires careful mobilization by removing scar tissue. The malleus, incus, and the prosthesis are carefully inspected and probed with a needle to assess their integrity and mobility. If soft tissue adhesions covering the middle ear structures are present, they are vaporized (Fig. 5.3 and Table 5.1).

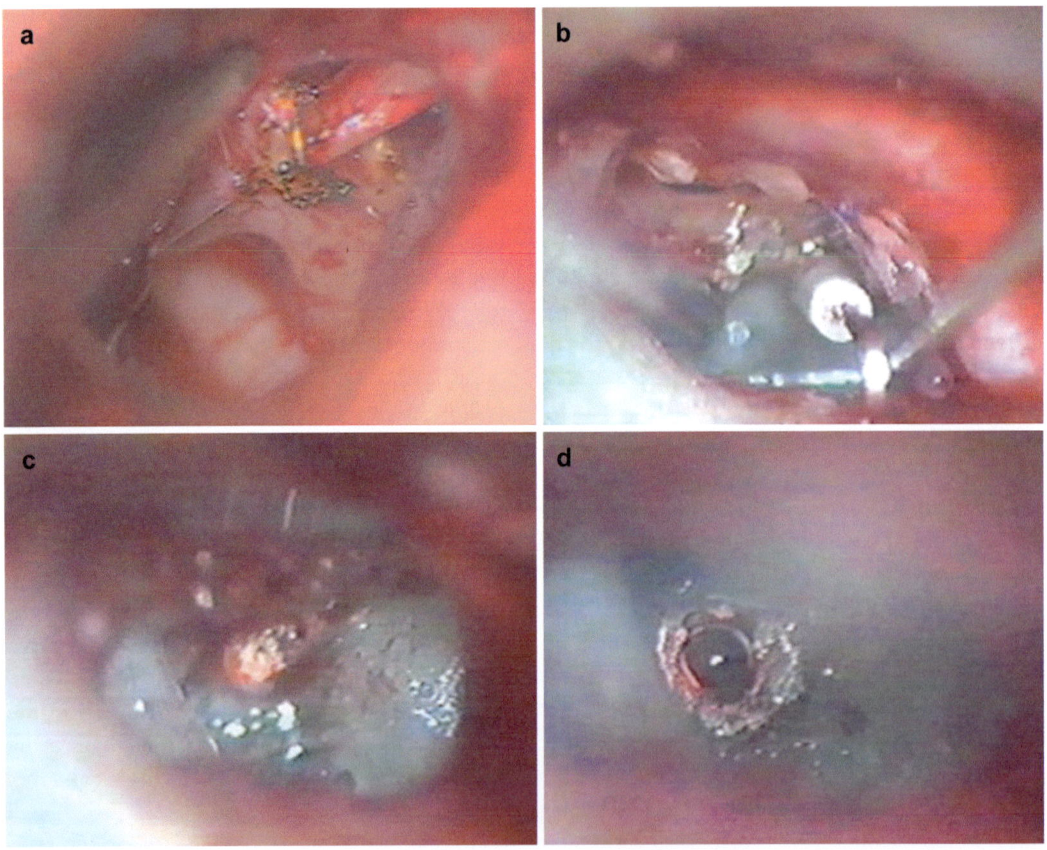

Fig. 5.3 (**a**) Stepwise exposure of the middle ear structures. (**b**) Extraction of the prosthesis. (**c**) Exposure of the oval niche. (**d**) Reperforated stapes footplate

5.3.2 Exposure of the Prosthesis and the Oval Niche

Connective tissue covering the prosthesis can be removed by laser vaporization (Fig. 5.3b). A power setting of 1–2 W and a pulse duration of 0.05 s are used to clean the oval window niche from connective and granulation tissue to visualize the margins of the footplate and to check if the piston is in the stapedotomy opening. To reduce mechanical trauma to the inner ear, only the laser should be used adhering to a noncontact technique. Next, the prosthesis is detached from the incus with a 2 mm long 90° hook and subsequently extracted. If, in the case of remaining parts of the stapes superstructure (e.g., posterior crus), bone needs to be vaporized, the laser is set to 6 W. Direct irradiation of the prosthesis should be minimized to reduce heat conduction to the inner ear. If the prosthesis contains Teflon components, direct laser irradiation of the prosthesis with 1–2 W can be regarded as safe; however, higher laser powers (e.g., >6 W) should be avoided since it has been observed that Teflon prostheses can be damaged by heat.

5.3.3 Re-perforation of the Stapes Footplate

Neo-membrane If the stapes footplate is covered with a connective tissue neo-membrane, a 4–8 W laser application with a pulse duration of 0.03–0.05 s, depending on the scanner diameter (0.4 mm, 0.5 mm, 0.6 mm), should be applied using the one-shot technique.

Bony footplate In the case of a bony footplate or if the preexisting perforation is too small (with or without membranous covering), a 20–22 W laser application with a pulse duration of 0.03–0.05 s can be applied with the scanner system using the one-shot technique.

Small existing perforation If the existing perforation is only slightly too small, an enlargement of the perforation can be achieved with multiple shots using a small focused laser beam (180 μm). Laser power of 1–2 W (membranous covering of the footplate) or 6–8 W (bony footplate) without using the scanner is applied in a slightly overlapping pattern (pulse duration of 0.05 s) to achieve an appropriate perforation (Fig. 5.2, middle, right).

Independently of the technique used, the tissue in the posterior part of the oval window should be uniformly vaporized to create a perforation of 0.5 mm (piston diameter of 0.4 mm) or 0.7 mm (piston diameter 0.6 mm) in diameter. After the laser procedure, vestibular perilymph should be visible through the opening in the foot plate. An irradiation of the empty vestibulum must be avoided in all cases (Fig. 5.3d).

Incus erosion If the incus is severely eroded, a malleovestibulopexy as described elsewhere should be performed to re-establish sound conduction.

Conclusion

Apart from convincing postoperative hearing results, the main advantage of the laser stapedotomy is that this technique can be safely applied in all cases of otosclerosis: early otosclerosis where the footplate is less fixed. Floating footplates after failed conventional stapedotomy can be treated as well as cases of obliterative otosclerosis or revision cases.

The combination of a CO_2 laser with a micromanipulator and a laser scanner is advantageous since a perforation can be achieved in most cases with a single shot.

References

1. Beatty TW, Haberkamp TJ, Khafagy YW, et al. Stapedectomy training with the carbon dioxide laser. Laryngoscope. 1997;107:1441–4.
2. Buchman CA, Fucci MJ, Roberson Jr JB, et al. Comparison of argon and CO2 laser stapedotomy in primary otosclerosis surgery. Am J Otolaryngol. 2000;21:227–30.
3. Dibartolomeo JR. The argon and CO2 lasers in otolaryngology: which one, when and why? Laryngoscope. 1981;91:1–16.

4. Fisch U, Acar GO, Huber AM. Malleostapedotomy in revision surgery for otosclerosis. Otol Neurotol. 2001;22:776–85.
5. Gersdorff M, Nouwen J, Gilain C, et al. Tinnitus and otosclerosis. Eur Arch Otorhinolaryngol. 2000;257: 314–6.
6. Gherini SG, Horn KL, Bowman CA, et al. Small fenestra stapedotomy using a fiberoptic hand-held argon laser in obliterative otosclerosis. Laryngoscope. 1990;100:1276–82.
7. Glasscock 3rd ME, Storper IS, Haynes DS, et al. Twenty-five years of experience with stapedectomy. Laryngoscope. 1995;105:899–904.
8. Hammerschlag PE, Fishman A, Scheer AA. A review of 308 cases of revision stapedectomy. Laryngoscope. 1998;108:1794–800.
9. Horn KL, Gherini SG, Franz DC. Argon laser revision stapedectomy. Am J Otol. 1994;15:383–8.
10. Hough JV, Dyer Jr RK. Stapedectomy. Causes of failure and revision surgery in otosclerosis. Otolaryngol Clin North Am. 1993;26:453–70.
11. Jovanovic S, Anft D, Schonfeld U, et al. Experimental studies on the suitability of the erbium laser for stapedotomy in an animal model. Eur Arch Otorhinolaryngol. 1995;252:422–7.
12. Jovanovic S, Anft D, Schonfeld U, et al. Influence of CO2 laser application to the guinea-pig cochlea on compound action potentials. Am J Otol. 1999;20: 166–73.
13. Jovanovic S, Jamali Y, Anft D, et al. Influence of pulsed laser irradiation on the morphology and function of the guinea pig cochlea. Hear Res. 2000;144:97–108.
14. Jovanovic S, Schonfeld U. Application of the CO2 laser in stapedotomy. Adv Otorhinolaryngol. 1995;49: 95–100.
15. Jovanovic S, Schonfeld U, Fischer R, et al. Thermal stress on the inner ear in laser stapedotomy. HNO. 1996;44:6–13.
16. Jovanovic S, Schonfeld U, Prapavat V, et al. Effects of continuous-wave laser systems on stapes footplate. Lasers Surg Med. 1996;19:424–32.
17. Jovanovic S, Schonfeld U, Scherer H. CO2 laser stapedotomy with the "one-shot" technique – clinical results. Otolaryngol Head Neck Surg. 2004;131:750–7.
18. Krieger LW, Lippy WH, Schuring AG, et al. Revision stapedectomy for incus erosion: long-term hearing. Otolaryngol Head Neck Surg. 1998;119:370–3.
19. Lesinski SG. Revision stapedectomy. Curr Opin Otolaryngol Head Neck Surg. 2003;11:347–54.
20. Lesinski SG, Newrock R. Carbon dioxide lasers for otosclerosis. Otolaryngol Clin North Am. 1993;26:417–41.
21. Lesinski SG, Palmer A. CO2 laser for otosclerosis: safe energy parameters. Laryngoscope. 1989;99: 9–12.
22. Lesinski SG, Stein JA. Stapedectomy revision with the CO2 laser. Laryngoscope. 1989;99:13–9.
23. Mcgee TM, Diaz-Ordaz EA, Kartush JM. The role of KTP laser in revision stapedectomy. Otolaryngol Head Neck Surg. 1993;109:839–43.
24. Oswal V, Remacle M, Jovanovic S, et al. Principles and Practice of Lasers in Otorhinolaryngology and Head and Neck Surgery-2nd Edition, Kugler Publications; Amsterdam, The Netherlands; 2014. p. 561–85.
25. Raman R, Mathew J, Idikula J. Obliterative otosclerosis. J Laryngol Otol. 1991;105:899–900.
26. Schmid P, Hausler R. Revision stapedectomy: an analysis of 201 operations. Otol Neurotol. 2009;30: 1092–100.
27. Shea Jr JJ. The teflon piston operation for otosclerosis. Laryngoscope. 1963;73:508–9.
28. Sheehy JL, Nelson RA, House HP. Revision stapedectomy: a review of 258 cases. Laryngoscope. 1981;91:43–51.
29. Sobrinho PG, Oliveira CA, Venosa AR. Long-term follow-up of tinnitus in patients with otosclerosis after stapes surgery. Int Tinnitus J. 2004;10: 197–201.
30. Szymanski M, Morshed K, Mills RP. The use of CO(2) laser in revision stapes surgery: experimental studies on heat transmission to the vestibule. Adv Otorhinolaryngol. 2007;65:250–4.
31. Wada H, Kobayashi T, Suetake M, et al. Dynamic behavior of the middle ear based on sweep frequency tympanometry. Audiology. 1989;28:127–34.
32. Wiet RJ, Kubek DC, Lemberg P, et al. A meta-analysis review of revision stapes surgery with argon laser: effectiveness and safety. Am J Otol. 1997;18:166–71.

6 Congenital Stapes Fixation

Joseph T. Breen, Matthew L. Carlson, and Colin L.W. Driscoll

6.1 Introduction

Conductive hearing loss (CHL) not related to otitis media affects only a small proportion of children with hearing impairment. Regardless of the cause, hearing loss has negative effects on language skills and intellectual development in children. The early diagnosis and appropriate treatment of congenital CHL in this population are therefore of the utmost importance.

The most commonly identified entities leading to fixation of the stapes footplate in children are congenital stapes footplate fixation (CSFF) and juvenile otosclerosis (JO) [1]. CSFF was first characterized by Shambaugh in 1952, when he differentiated the entity from otosclerosis as a nonprogressive conductive loss noted since birth, with an unremarkable family history and a fixed stapes footplate seen at the time of surgery. He presented five such cases, which were all treated by lateral canal fenestration [2]. Since then, the body of knowledge regarding middle ear malformations and outcomes after surgery for CSFF has grown slowly, but the optimal form of treatment is still a matter of controversy.

6.1.1 Pathophysiology

The stapes primarily develops from the second branchial arch, with the exception of its medial inner lamina of the footplate and the annular ligament, which are derived from the otic capsule. The malleus and incus are believed to be of both first and second branchial arch origin, with the head of the malleus and body of the incus deriving from the first arch and the long process of the incus and the manubrium of the malleus deriving from the second arch [3]. In some cases of footplate fixation, particularly those with syndromic associations, several of the second arch derivatives are abnormal. Abnormalities of ossicular second arch derivatives are more common than first arch derivatives, and they most commonly occur in isolation without other second arch abnormalities elsewhere in the head and neck. No clear explanation for this pattern has been presented [4].

A long-standing theory of the pathophysiology of isolated congenital footplate fixation is the lack of differentiation of the peripheral lamina stapedialis into the annular ligament [5]. At the time of surgery, this may appear as a diffusely thickened white footplate. Many other stapes and

J.T. Breen, MD (✉)
Department of Otolaryngology – Head and Neck Surgery, Baylor College of Medicine, Houston, TX, USA
e-mail: jbreen@bcm.edu

M.L. Carlson, MD • C.L.W. Driscoll, MD
Department of Otorhinolaryngology – Head and Neck Surgery, Mayo Clinic, Rochester, MN, USA
e-mail: carlson.matthew@mayo.edu; driscoll.colin@mayo.edu

I. Sziklai (ed.), *Surgery of Stapes Fixations*, DOI 10.1007/978-3-319-28576-4_6

footplate abnormalities seen at the time of middle ear exploration have been reported, including ossified stapedial tendon [6], malpositioned, malformed, or absent stapes crura [7–9], narrow oval window niche, obliterated obturator foramen [8], confluent oval and round windows [10], and prolapsed, bifid, or aberrant facial nerve [11]. These can occur in isolation, in combination with footplate fixation, or in combination with other ossicular abnormalities. Malformations of the footplate can occur along a continuum, with the most severe form being complete absence of the stapes and oval window.

Otosclerosis is the abnormal reabsorption and deposition of otic capsule bone and most commonly only becomes symptomatic when this process leads to fixation of the stapes footplate. Its relevant anatomy and pathophysiology are more fully discussed elsewhere in this text. Juvenile otosclerosis, by definition, is the occurrence of this process in patients under 18 years of age. Histologic temporal bone studies have shown that otosclerosis is relatively uncommon in the very young, with less than 0.6 % of temporal bones showing evidence of the disease before the age of 5 and 4 % of those between 5 and 18 years [12]. Similar cadaveric and clinical studies find an 8.3–13.7 % rate of the disease in adult Caucasian ears [13]. Though it is atypical for otosclerosis to clinically manifest early in life, it should be recognized that overall the disease process is more prevalent than CSFF in children.

6.1.2 Epidemiology

Congenital hearing loss due to ossicular anomalies is uncommon. A published estimate of the rate of congenital ear anomalies in general is 1 in 15,000, and only a subset of these will involve the middle ear [14]. In most series of patients with congenital CHL, fixation of the stapes footplate is the most common isolated ossicular abnormality encountered at the time of middle ear exploration. Park and colleagues [4] reported a group of 78 South Korean patients with normal auricles and tympanic membranes who underwent middle ear explorations and were found to have ossicular malformations. Of these, 53 (68 %) had stapes footplate fixation, and in 36 (46 %), this was an isolated anomaly with an otherwise normal ossicular chain. Interestingly, they reported that when stapes footplate fixation was isolated abnormality, it was found to be in both ears 86 % of the time. When CSFF occurred in conjunction with another ossicular abnormality (ten patients), it was always unilateral.

Teunissen and Cremers [9] proposed a classification system for congenital middle ear abnormalities when they reviewed their operated congenital CHL cases in 1993. In their series of 144 operated ears with congenital ossicular abnormalities, 44 (30 %) had isolated CSFF – the most commonly seen isolated abnormality. An additional 55 (38 %) patients had another ossicular abnormality in conjunction with footplate fixation. Only 31 (22 %) had any other ossicular abnormality without footplate fixation. Congenital oval window aplasia or dysplasia was seen in an additional 14 patients (10 %).

6.2 Diagnosis

6.2.1 History

For children with CHL, some key elements of patient history can help narrow the differential diagnosis. A significant history of chronic otitis media should raise suspicion for effusion, tympanosclerosis, acquired ossicular abnormalities, or cholesteatoma. Additionally, children with atretic ears have an obvious cause for CHL, though a sizable portion of these patients will also have comorbid ossicular malformations, which can include footplate fixation. In the absence of these more obvious diagnoses, is critical to elucidate whether the hearing deficit was potentially present since birth. In many cases, the loss will not be recognized for years. Children with significant loss may develop lip reading skills and fail to realize or alert their caregivers to the presence of the deficit [15]. Even if a firm diagnosis is not obtained in the first years of life, the clinician should maintain a high degree of suspicion that the loss is congenital.

If normal hearing is clearly documented early in life or the older child can reliably provide a history of progressive loss, a diagnosis of JO should be considered. However, this is often difficult to accurately sort out. House and colleagues [15] first highlighted that CSFF and JO can be differentiated from one another primarily by eliciting this history of progression.

Family history can further help identify those with JO, as otosclerosis seems to have the strongest genetic element of the disease processes leading to footplate fixation. Family cohorts with CSFF have been reported, however. Patients with progressive conductive or mixed hearing loss with features consistent with X-linked recessive inheritance (only males affected) should raise the question of X-linked congenital mixed hearing loss and X-linked gusher syndrome [16].

6.2.2 Physical Exam

Patients with CSFF will commonly have normal physical examinations. As with all patients with hearing loss, a complete head and neck exam should be performed, including assessment of cranial nerve function, tuning fork testing, pneumatic otoscopy, and binocular otomicroscopy when possible.

The presence of craniofacial dysmorphisms and auricular malformations that do not seem to account for the degree of conductive loss should strongly point towards a congenital ossicular abnormality. Multiple syndromes can include stapes footplate fixations or other ossicular abnormalities, including branchio-oto-renal syndrome, Goldenhar (oculo-auriculo-vertebral) syndrome, and Teunissen-Cremers syndrome (stapes fixation, severe hyperopia, and phalangeal abnormalities).

6.2.3 Audiometry

Further information to differentiate CSFF from JO can be garnered from the audiogram. House noted that CSFF generally presented with a flat air conduction curve with a three tone PTA of approximately 50 dB. Additionally, the bone line would remain within the 0–10 dB threshold range. The audiometric configuration of JO was more variable, with a lesser degree of conductive loss in most patients. They posited that once the degree of conductive loss exceeded 35 dB, the diagnosis of CSFF was more likely. Additionally, patients with JO are more likely to demonstrate a Carhart notch at 2 kHz than are those with CSFF [17]. These audiometric characteristics are represented graphically in Fig. 6.1. As with all cases of

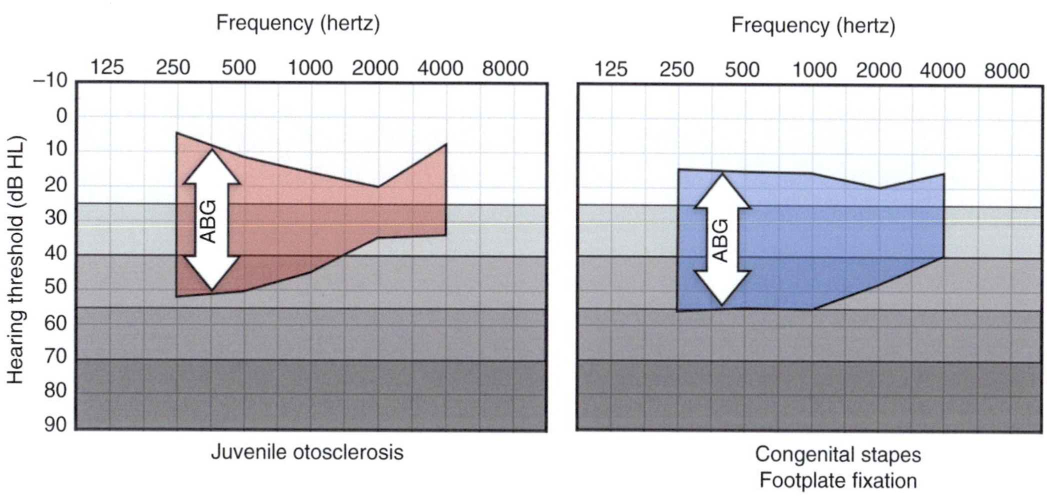

Fig. 6.1 Typical audiometric characteristics for juvenile otosclerosis and congenital stapes footplate fixation. CSFF tends to present with a flatter and more significant impairment, with a less prominent Carhart notch when compared to JO (Reprinted with permission from Carlson et al. [17])

ossicular fixation, stapes reflexes are expected to be absent with all processes that lead to pediatric footplate fixation.

6.2.4 Imaging

All children suspected of having stapes footplate fixation should undergo high-resolution CT scanning of the temporal bones before surgery. CT may identify the etiology of the hearing loss, which can aid in surgical planning and counseling patients and parents regarding expectations with surgery. However, even modern high-resolution scans are often unable to clearly show pathology at the footplate that is seen at the time of surgery [12]. A normal appearing scan should not be seen as a contraindication to exploration.

Most relevant to the patient with congenital hearing loss, inner ear malformations can be identified on preoperative imaging. Most view this as a strict contraindication to opening the vestibule due to heightened risk of postoperative SNHL. Visualization of a patent round window and normal oval window-facial nerve relationship can also be helpful in making the decision to offer surgery [1].

6.3 Treatment

6.3.1 Amplification

For almost all patients with conductive or mixed hearing loss, hearing aids are a viable option for treatment, and patients with congenital conductive loss are no exception to this. Young children with clinically significant bilateral hearing impairment should be fitted for hearing aids once diagnosed. A suggested degree of hearing loss for considering amplification is a speech reception threshold of 30 dB HL [18]. The utility of aiding children with unilateral hearing loss is not universally agreed upon, but a significant body of data exists to suggest that children with unilateral hearing loss tend to have more difficulty in school and worse language skills [19]. Improvements in multiple quality of life domains have been demonstrated after amplification in school age children with unilateral hearing loss [20]. Sound localization improvements after unilateral amplification have been shown to be greater in younger children, suggesting a role of central hearing pathway development with earlier noise exposure [21]. In situations of unilateral hearing impairment, the benefits should be explained to the patient and family members to allow them to adequately weigh the relative pros and cons of a hearing aid.

6.3.2 Informed Consent and Perioperative Care

When the relatively effective and low-risk alternative of conventional amplification exists, decision-making regarding elective surgery can be challenging. Legal medical decision-making will usually rest with the parents or other family members for individuals under 18 in many countries. Many children will clearly have the capacity to discuss and consider the relative merits of surgery before this age, however, and there will be a joint decision-making process that includes the patient's wishes. Some surgeons may choose to wait until a child can participate in this process before offering a middle ear exploration. Finally, delaying should decrease the probability that surgery will be complicated by otitis media or effusion. A combination of these factors leads most surgeons to delay until at least the age of 5 before considering an operation [22].

Some reports have suggested that earlier surgical intervention may be in the best interest of children with JO. Their early age of presentation may be predictive of obliterative disease that would require a drill-out if it was allowed to progress. This additional caveat should be considered when weighing treatment options for the young patient with progressive CHL potentially due to JO [23].

6.3.3 Surgery

Stapes surgery has evolved significantly over the past 60 years. Refinements in surgical technique and prostheses have led to consistently excellent rates of air bone gap (ABG) closure with low complication rates in many large series [24]. Despite this vast body of knowledge, there is a relative paucity of data regarding stapes surgery in children. Earlier reports of relatively unfavorable outcomes and complications coupled with a desire for non-maleficence when treating children significantly tempered enthusiasm for operating on patients with suspected CSFF. This hesitance combined with the relative rarity of the condition leads to there being only a handful of publications that have reviewed outcomes after surgery for CSFF.

If the pathology is found to be isolated to the stapes footplate at the time of middle ear exploration, stapedectomy or small fenestra stapedotomy is likely to be the treatment of choice. Surgical techniques and prostheses used for patients in larger published case series are heterogeneous. Transcanal approaches are utilized by many [17, 25], but endaural [12, 25] and postauricular approaches are also used as a matter of surgeon preference. Authors from an earlier report of surgery for CSFF advocated for a postauricular approach in cases of congenital CHL, backed by the rationale that if malleus fixation is encountered, the access required for correction will be available [15]. It should be noted that this was before the era of CT scanning, and hence it would be difficult to isolate the problem to the footplate preoperatively. Conversion to a postauricular approach may be necessary in some cases to provide adequate exposure. The degree of footplate removal ranges in the literature from small fenestra stapedotomy to partial footplate removal or complete stapedectomy.

For patients with otosclerosis, stapes mobilization is not first-line surgical treatment. The continuous remodeling of otic capsule bone is not altered by the procedure, and ultimately this can lead to refixation of the stapes footplate with reversal of the gains in hearing obtained with the procedure. CSFF is a developmental anomaly that should not be associated with abnormal bone turnover later in life. As such, some have proposed that the relatively less invasive stapes mobilization procedure should be considered with CSFF, as refixation should be less likely in these patients [26]. In the event that a patient has a history clearly compatible with CSFF and a simple mobilization is possible, it can be considered. Syms and De la Cruz [27] reported a preference for stapes mobilization in cases of CSFF when the footplate was cartilaginous in appearance. However, the degree of bony fixation at the footplate may be extensive in CSFF, with a continuum of abnormalities ranging all the way to complete agenesis of the oval window, where mobilization is obviously not a possibility.

6.3.4 Results

One of the first reports of results from surgery for congenital footplate fixation was published in 1958, when Howard House and colleagues [15] attempted mobilization procedures by "needle and chisel techniques" on 23 patients with CSFF ranging from 6 to 60 years of age, with an average of 33 years. Twelve (52 %) of their patients experienced an improvement of 11 dB or more in their air conduction pure tone average, with the remainder unchanged. Five were unable to be mobilized and three of these subsequently underwent lateral canal fenestration with resultant improvement to an air conduction PTA of 30 dB HL or better. The length of follow-up was not reported, but no cases of refixation were seen in the subset of patients who were seen back 1 year after surgery. An update to this report with more patients and longer (though still not well characterized) follow-up in 1969 stated that 6 of the 23 mobilized ears that showed initial hearing gains subsequently showed evidence of refixation [28].

In subsequent years, surgeons began attempting interventions other than stapes mobilization or fenestration in cases of CSFF with variable results. The majority of surgeons publishing on the matter come to the conclusion that stapedotomy or stapedectomy on ears with CSFF is generally safe, but many find their audiometric outcomes to be less satisfactory than those achieved for otosclerosis [1, 4, 7–9, 17, 25, 29–36]. A sampling of the literature to date with adequate audiometric data and length of follow-up regarding outcomes after surgery for CSFF is presented in Table 6.1.

Table 6.1 Surgical outcomes for congenital stapes fixation

Publication	# of cases	Age (range, median, mean)	Pre-PTA	Pre-ABG	Post-PTA	Post-ABG	PTA gain	Post-op SN loss >10 dB (#, %)	Post-op profound SN Loss (#, %)	Post-op ABG <10	Post-op ABG <20	Post-op ABG <30	Follow-up (mean)
Carlson 2013	27	5.7–18.9, 15.3, 13.8	51.7	34.1	32.8	17.2	18.9	1 (4 %)	0	9 (33 %)	21 (78 %)	23 (85 %)	43 months
Denoyelle 2010	25							0	0	17 (68 %)	25 (100 %)	25 (100 %)	2 months
Thomeer 2010	39	9–27, x, 15.3	46	36	25	14	21	1 (3 %)	0	18 (46 %)	29 (74 %)		12 months
Park 2009	56							NR	NR		40 (71 %)		
Albert 2006	28	8.3–29.1, 14.2, ?	50.0	35.0	15.0	10.0	35.0	0	0				12 months
Massey 2006	25	6–71, 14				12.2		2 (8 %)	0	12 (48 %)	20 (80 %)		
Bachor 2005	6	7–13, 9, 9.3	51.4	35	44.7	21	6.7	3 (50 %)	0	1 (17 %)	3 (50 %)	5 (83 %)	0.75–12 months
Welling, 2003	21		42.8	33.2	21.7	21.1	21.1	0	0	5 (24 %)	14 (67 %)	NR	27.8 months
Raveh 2002	12							1 (8 %)	1 (8 %)	2 (17 %)	3 (25 %)	4 (33 %)	
Hashimoto 2002	23		52	31	28	9	24	0	0		21 (91 %)		
De la Cruz 1999	44	11.4 (mean)	55.1	35.2				0	0	44 %			
Dornhoffer 1995	10	6–16, 8, 9	52.8	37.4	27.7	10.9	25.1	0	0	5 (50 %)	9 (90 %)	10 (100 %)	6–12 months
Teunissen 1990	32		55		37		20	4 (13 %)	2 (6 %)	18 (56 %)	23 (72 %)	27 (84 %)	1–19 years, avg 5 years
House 1980	13	4.5–17						1 (8 %)	1 (8 %)	10 (77 %)			
Funasaka 1979	7	6–38, 9, 16	65.6		58.1		7.5	2 (29 %)	1 (14 %)				6 months

Summary of selected publications reviewing hearing outcomes after surgery for congenital stapes fixation

In 1980, John House et al. [34] presented a series of 34 children with CHL that underwent middle ear exploration; 20 of these were found to have congenital fixation of the stapes footplate. They proceeded with stapedectomy or a drill-out procedure on 13 patients in this subset. One patient (who was one of the three that underwent a drill-out) was found to have a dead ear postoperatively. Ten patients closed their ABG to within 10 dB. They additionally presented a group of ears with JO who underwent stapedectomy; 22 of 24 closed their ABG to 10 dB or less, though again one patient developed profound SNHL. This led the group to conclude that stapedectomy can be performed on children with satisfactory results.

Von Haacke [37] reported his experience in 1985 with a less optimistic view on surgery for CSFF. Two patients with CSFF underwent surgery, with one patient developing a significant SNHL postoperatively and the other being left with a significant CHL. They additionally explored outcomes after stapes surgery in the setting of osteogenesis imperfecta (OI) and tympanosclerosis, ultimately concluding that stapes surgery for conditions other than otosclerosis and perhaps OI is potentially not advisable.

Dornhoffer [33] reported results from ten ears (seven patients) that underwent small fenestra stapedotomy for congenital footplate fixation. Of these, 5 (50 %) achieved ABG closure to less than 10 dB, 9 (90 %) to within 20 dB, and one patient was left with a persistent 25 dB ABG. No cases were complicated by perilymph gusher or worsening of their air conduction thresholds postoperatively.

Hashimoto et al. [38] reported a 91 % rate (21 of 23 ears) of closing the ABG to less than 20 dB with an improvement of at least 15 dB in the air conduction PTA for patients with congenital CHL and stapes fixation. Additionally, two of four additional patients who had stapes footplate fixation with incudostapedial joint abnormalities underwent a successful surgery. The majority (19) of these patients underwent small fenestra stapedotomy, with two undergoing stapes mobilization and the remainder undergoing total stapedectomy. Patients with incudostapedial joint abnormalities underwent either ossiculoplasty with cortical bone (three patients) or malleus to vestibule reconstruction with a piston wire (one patient). No patients had worsening of their hearing after surgery.

Welling and colleagues [31] reported a series of 66 ears that underwent stapes surgery, with 21 of these carrying a diagnosis of CSFF. Of these, five ears (24 %) demonstrated a postoperative ABG of <10 dB, an additional nine ears (43 %) had a postoperative ABG between 10 and 20 dB, and the remainder (seven ears, 33 %) were left with an ABG of greater than 20 dB. They reported no cases of profound hearing loss postoperatively.

Most recently, Carlson et al. [17] presented their experience with pediatric stapes surgery, including 27 operated ears with CSFF. The average residual ABG after was 17.2 dB, with an average improvement in air conduction PTA of 18.9 dB. When compared to the pediatric cohort that underwent surgery for JO, the average postoperative ABG was significantly poorer in the CSFF group (mean 17.2 dB vs. 8.8 dB; $p=0.04$). While not universally reported, this tendency towards worse outcomes for CSFF as compared to JO has been corroborated by several other surgeons.

Not surprisingly, the severity of the malformation seen at the time of surgery seems to be inversely correlated to the probability of a successful outcome. Park and Choung [4] published a large series of patients with a wide variety of isolated ossicular abnormalities that underwent middle ear exploration and attempted correction. Of their 94 ears (78 patients), 63 ears had abnormalities of the stapes or stapes footplate fixation. None of the seven ears that had congenitally absent stapes footplates had good results (residual ABG of <20 dB) in their series. Additionally, only 30 % (3 of 10) patients who had stapes footplate fixation combined with any other ossicular abnormality (including malformations of the stapes) had a good outcome, as compared to 80.4 % (37 of 46) of ears with CSFF alone. Funasaka [35] noticed a similar correlation in his small series, reporting deterioration of hearing in the two of the seven operated ears with CSFF where the oval window was maldeveloped. Jahrsdoerfer [6] reported that his subset of congenitally absent oval window (CAOW) patients did relatively well, however, with four of six closing their ABG to 20 dB or less after labyrinthotomy and prosthesis placement and no patients losing hearing. A summary of published reports of results after surgery for congenitally absent oval window can be found in Table 6.2 [4, 6, 39, 40]. On average, modest increases in hearing can be seen after surgery for CAOW, with most patients still left with ABGs larger than those usually seen after surgery for isolated CSFF. In some reports, the gains in hearing were often partially lost over time [39].

6.3.5 Complications

One of the most feared complications of any surgery for footplate fixation is SNHL. In most modern series, the rate of significant new sensorineural loss after stapes surgery approximates 1 % [24]. Some reports suggesting a significantly increased chance of this complication led some surgeons to advise against stapedotomy or stapedectomy for patients with CSFF [1].

When results from several reports of surgery for CSFF are compiled (Table 6.1), it appears that significant postoperative hearing loss occurs rarely – not markedly more frequently than it does in surgery for otosclerosis. When taken in aggregate, there were five cases of profound (>80 dB) SNHL after surgery after CSFF among 305 operated ears for which adequate data was reported – a rate of 1.6 %. There were a total of 15 cases (4.9 %) where the bone conduction PTA dropped more than 10 dB postoperatively in this group.

Copious cerebrospinal fluid (CSF) otorrhea (or perilymph "gusher") during stapes surgery has been seen during surgery for both otosclerosis as well as for congenital footplate fixation and is seen at much higher rates in patients with inner ear anomalies. Several routes for this anomalous route of CSF egress have been suggested [5, 41]. The cochlear aqueduct is a bony channel between the basal turn of the cochlea and the posterior fossa. It transmits the periotic duct, which allows communication between scala tympani and the subarachnoid space. It has been posited that an unusually patent cochlear aqueduct could be a route by which CSF flows through the opened footplate in cases of perilymph gusher. A more commonly held theory, however, is that abnormal patency at the fundus of the internal auditory canal that communicates with the perilymphatic space. The periotic space surrounding the endolymphatic duct has also been suggested as a route but has not been well substantiated [5].

The occurrence of a perilymph gusher at the time of stapes surgery is not always associated with a significant postoperative SNHL. Indeed, several reports have demonstrated adequate hearing outcomes after being appropriately managed interoperatively with some form of tissue graft to form a seal around the prosthesis. Dornhoffer pointed out that a preoperative SNHL superimposed upon the conductive loss may be predictive of worsening of hearing when a gusher is encountered, however [33].

Prolapsed or anomalous facial nerve courses can be seen in patients with footplate abnormalities or other middle ear pathologies, and this can significantly impact surgical decision-making. In particular, the facial nerve course is most likely to be aberrant in cases of oval window dysplasia or absence [6, 39, 42]. De Alarcon et al. noted that ten of their 17 patients who underwent an attempted drill-out for congenitally absent oval window (CAOW) had abnormal facial nerve courses in the middle ear. Su et al. [40] similarly reported that 67 of 97 patients who underwent surgery for CAOW had facial nerve course abnormalities. It has been suggested that perhaps an abnormally anterior course of the facial nerve disrupts the normal contact between the otic capsule and stapes blastema during development, leading to malformation of both of these structures [42]. Most commonly seen facial nerve abnormalities relevant to surgery for CSFF or CAOW include partial or complete obstruction of the oval window, dehiscent facial nerve, bifid nerve that is split around the stapes and oval window, and displacement of the nerve anterior and inferior to the oval window (Fig. 6.2). Facial nerve injury during surgery for congenital stapes

Table 6.2 Congenital absence of the oval window

Publication	# of cases	Age (range, median, mean)	Pre-PTA	Pre-ABG	Post-PTA	Post-ABG	PTA gain	SN loss >10 dB (#, %)	Post-op ABG <10	Post-op ABG <20	Post-op ABG <30	Follow-up (mean)
Park 2009	7							NR	0 (0 %)	0 (0 %)		6 months
Yu Su 2014	56	6–31, x, 15.7	67	50	49	31	18	0				
De Alarcon 2008	13	5–20, x, 9	61	49	43	31	18	0				
Jahrsdoerfer 1980	6							0	1 (17 %)	4 (67 %)	5 (83 %)	

Summary of selected publications reviewing hearing outcomes after surgery for congenital absence of the oval window

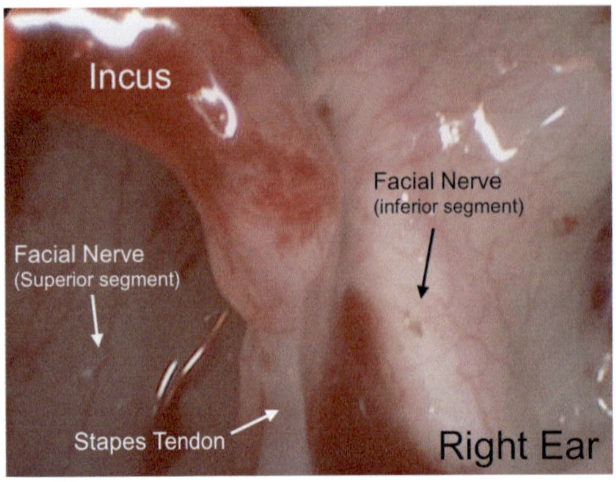

Fig. 6.2 The stapes suprastructure is malformed, with an aberrant bifid facial nerve coursing above and below the oval window

or footplate abnormalities is infrequently reported, but abnormalities in its course can lead the surgeon to abort surgery.

Conclusion

Congenital fixation of the stapes footplate is a rare but distinct clinical entity that presents the otologist with a unique set of challenges. Congenital abnormalities of the stapes footplate can vary in severity, and when additional middle and inner ear malformations are also present, postoperative hearing outcomes are generally slightly poorer than stapedectomy for otosclerosis and the risks of complications can be higher. Preoperative imaging should be obtained in all cases of suspected congenital CHL to help the surgeon and patient prepare for these possibilities. Thorough counseling of patients and their parents regarding the risks and benefits of surgery is important, and amplification should be recommended to all children with bilateral congenital CHL (SRT >30 dB HL) as soon as the deficit is identified. In properly selected patients, surgery has an acceptable risk profile, but it has been the experience of many surgeons that hearing outcomes are often inferior to those seen with surgery for otosclerosis.

References

1. De la Cruz A, Angeli S, Slattery WH. Stapedectomy in children. Otolaryngol Head Neck Surg Off J Am Acad Otolaryngol Head Neck Surg. 1999;120(4):487–92. doi:10.1053/hn.1999.v120.a89626.
2. Shambaugh GE. Developmental anomalies of the sound conducting apparatus and their surgical correction. Trans Am Otological Soc. 1952;40:217–31.
3. Gulya AJ. Anatomy of the temporal bone with surgical implications. 3rd ed. CRC Press; Informa Healthcare, New York, NY 2007.
4. Park K, Choung Y-H. Isolated congenital ossicular anomalies. Acta Otolaryngol. 2009;129(4):419–22. doi:10.1080/00016480802587846.
5. Olson NR, Lehman RH. Cerebrospinal fluid otorrhea and the congenitally fixed stapes. Laryngoscope. 1968;78(3):352–60. doi: 10.1288/00005537-196803000-00006.
6. Jahrsdoerfer R. Congenital malformations of the ear. Analysis of 94 operations. Ann Otol Rhinol Laryngol. 1980;89(4 Pt 1):348–52.
7. Albert S, Roger G, Rouillon I, Chauvin P, Denoyelle F, Derbez R, Delattre J, Triglia J-M, Garabedian E-N. Congenital stapes ankylosis: study of 28 cases and surgical results. Laryngoscope. 2006;116(7):1153–7. doi:10.1097/01.mlg.0000227501.78004.f6.
8. Bachor E, Just T, Wright CG, Pau HW, Karmody CS. Fixation of the stapes footplate in children: a clinical and temporal bone histopathologic study. Otol Neurotol Off Publ Am Otological Soc Am Neurotol Soc Eur Acad Otol Neurotol. 2005;26(5):866–73.
9. Teunissen EB, Cremers WR. Classification of congenital middle ear anomalies. Report on 144 ears. Ann Otol Rhinol Laryngol. 1993;102(8 Pt 1):606–12.
10. Cousins VC, Milton CM. Congenital ossicular abnormalities: a review of 68 cases. The American Journal of Otology. 1988;9(1):76–80
11. McRackan TR, Carlson ML, Reda FA, Noble JH, Rivas A. Bifid facial nerve in congenital stapes footplate fixation. Otol Neurotol Off Publ Am Otol Soc Am Neurotol Soc Eur Acad Otol Neurotol. 2014;35(5):e199–201. doi:10.1097/MAO.0000000000000274.
12. Lescanne E, Bakhos D, Metais JP, Robier A, Moriniere S. Otosclerosis in children and adolescents: a clinical and CT-scan survey with review of the literature. Int J Pediatr Otorhinolaryngol. 2008;72(2):147–52. doi:10.1016/j.ijporl.2007.10.017.
13. McKenna MJ, Merchant SN. Disorders of Bone. In: Merchant SN, Nadol JB, eds. Schunknecht's Pathology of the Ear. 3rd ed. Shelton, CT: PMPH-USA; 2010.
14. Farrior JB. Surgical management of congenital conductive deafness. South Med J. 1987;80(4):450–3.
15. House HP, House WF, Hildyard VH. Congenital stapes footplate fixation; a preliminary report of twenty-three

operated cases. Laryngoscope. 1958;68(8):1389–402. doi:10.1288/00005537-195808000-00003.
16. Teunissen B, Cremers WR, Huygen PL, Pouwels TP. Isolated congenital stapes ankylosis: surgical results in 32 ears and a review of the literature. Laryngoscope. 1990;100(12):1331–6. doi:10.1288/00005537-199012000-00017.
17. Carlson ML, Van Abel KM, Pelosi S, Beatty CW, Haynes DS, Wanna GB, Bennett ML, Driscoll CL. Outcomes comparing primary pediatric stapedectomy for congenital stapes footplate fixation and juvenile otosclerosis. Otol Neurotol Off Publ Am Otol Soc Am Neurotol Soc Eur Acad Otol Neurotol. 2013;34(5):816–20. doi:10.1097/MAO.0b013e318280db7b.
18. Stewart JM, Downs MP. Congenital conductive hearing loss: the need for early identification and intervention. Pediatrics. 1993;91(2):355–9.
19. Lieu JEC, Tye-Murray N, Fu Q. Longitudinal study of children with unilateral hearing loss. Laryngoscope. 2012;122(9):2088–95. doi:10.1002/lary.23454.
20. Briggs L, Davidson L, Lieu JEC. Outcomes of conventional amplification for pediatric unilateral hearing loss. Ann Otol Rhinol Laryngol. 2011;120(7):448–54.
21. Johnstone PM, Náběelek AK, Robertson VS. Sound localization acuity in children with unilateral hearing loss who wear a hearing aid in the impaired ear. J Am Acad Audiol. 2010;21(8):522–34. doi:10.3766/jaaa.21.8.4.
22. Briggs RJ, Luxford WM. Correction of conductive hearing loss in children. Otolaryngol Clin N Am. 1994;27(3):607–20.
23. Robinson M. Juvenile otosclerosis. A 20-year study. Ann Otol Rhinol Laryngol. 1983;92(6 Pt 1):561–5.
24. Vincent R, Sperling NM, Oates J, Jindal M. Surgical findings and long-term hearing results in 3,050 stapedotomies for primary otosclerosis: a prospective study with the otology-neurotology database. Otol Neurotol Off Publ Am Otol Soc Am Neurotol Soc Eur Acad Otol Neurotol. 2006;27(8 Suppl 2):S25–47. doi:10.1097/01.mao.0000235311.80066.df.
25. Thomeer HGXM, Kunst HPM, Cremers CWRJ. Congenital stapes ankylosis associated with another ossicular chain anomaly: surgical results in 30 ears. Arch Otolaryngol Head Neck Surg. 2011;137(9):935–41. doi:10.1001/archoto.2011.137.
26. Thiel G, Mills R. Rosen mobilization of the stapes: does it have a place in modern otology? J Laryngol Otol. 2006;120(12):1067–71. doi:10.1017/S0022215106002490.
27. Syms CA, De la Cruz A. Pediatric otology. Otolaryngol Clin N Am. 1996;29(3):407–20.
28. Steele BC. Congenital fixation of the stapes footplate. Acta Oto-Laryngologica. 1969;245:21–24.
29. Denoyelle F, Daval M, Leboulanger N, Rousseau A, Roger G, Loundon N, Rouillon I, Garabedian E-N. Stapedectomy in children: causes and surgical results in 35 cases. Arch Otolaryngol Head Neck Surg. 2010;136(10):1005–8. doi:10.1001/archoto.2010.170.
30. Massey B, Hillman T, Shelton C. Stapedectomy in congenital stapes fixation: are hearing outcomes poorer? Otolaryngol Head Neck Surg Off J Am Acad Otolaryngol Head Neck Surg. 2006;134(5):816–8. doi:10.1016/j.otohns.2005.10.063.
31. Welling DB, Merrell JA, Merz M, Dodson EE. Predictive factors in pediatric stapedectomy. Laryngoscope. 2003;113(9):1515–9. doi:10.1097/00005537-200309000-00018.
32. Raveh E, Hu W, Papsin BC, Forte V. Congenital conductive hearing loss. J Laryngol Otol. 2002; 116(2):92–6.
33. Dornhoffer JL, Helms J, Hoehmann DH. Stapedectomy for congenital fixation of the stapes. Am J Otol. 1995;16(3):382–6.
34. House JW, Sheehy JL, Antunez JC. Stapedectomy in children. Laryngoscope. 1980;90(11 Pt 1):1804–9.
35. Funasaka S. Congenital ossicular anomalies without malformations of the external ear. Arch Otol Rhinol Laryngol 1979;224(3–4):231–40.
36. Thomeer HGXM, Kunst HPM, Cremers CWRJ. Isolated congenital stapes ankylosis: surgical results in a consecutive series of 39 ears. Ann Otol Rhinol Laryngol. 2010;119(11):761–6.
37. von Haacke NP. Juvenile stapedectomy. Clin Otolaryngol Allied Sci. 1985;10(1):9–13.
38. Hashimoto S, Yamamoto Y, Satoh H, Takahashi S. Surgical treatment of 52 cases of auditory ossicular malformations. Auris Nasus Larynx. 2002;29(1):15–8.
39. de Alarcon A, Jahrsdoerfer RA, Kesser BW. Congenital absence of the oval window: diagnosis, surgery, and audiometric outcomes. Otol Neurotol Off Publ Am Otol Soc Am Neurotol Soc Eur Acad Otol Neurotol. 2008;29(1):23–8. doi:10.1097/mao.0b013e31815dbb28.
40. Su Y, Yuan H, Song Y-S, Shen W-D, Han W-J, Liu J, Han D-Y, Dai P. Congenital middle ear abnormalities with absence of the oval window: diagnosis, surgery, and audiometric outcomes. Otol Neurotol Off Publ Am Otol Soc Am Neurotol Soc Eur Acad Otol Neurotol. 2014;35(7):1191–5. doi:10.1097/MAO.0000000000000277.
41. Glasscock ME. The stapes gusher. Arch Otolaryngol (Chicago, Ill: 1960). 1973;98(2):82–91.
42. Lambert PR. Congenital absence of the oval window. Laryngoscope. 1990;100(1):37–40. doi:10.1288/00005537-199001000-00009.

7 Intraoperative Complications in Stapedectomy/Stapedotomy

O. Nuri Ozgirgin

7.1 Introduction

Stapes operation directed to repair the hearing loss due to the otosclerosis is believed to be technically difficult and bears challenges. So it has always been matter of discussion whether to let the residents perform the surgery or not. Even within the hands of experienced surgeons, the risk of sensorineural hearing loss rises up to 3 % (0.6–3 %) [1]. Even if the risk for other complications such as facial nerve impairment or further conductive hearing loss exists, they are negligible for the experienced surgeons.

Guyot and Sakbeni [2] recall myopia as there is still possible to wear glasses instead of surgery if the risk of total blindness of 1% in surgery makes the patient reluctant to give written consent. The authors focus on two patients' psychiatric problems having total hearing loss and long-term dizziness after stapedectomy. Even if the patients can adapt to the new condition, a great effort is needed for professional, family, mental, and emotional adaptation.

As considered systematically, the intratympanic complications will be discussed in regard to the surgical steps of stapes surgery.

The primary surgery is now conducted most often under general anesthesia. It is important for the anesthesiologist to offer hypotensive anesthesia during the surgery. Even if the patient is under general anesthesia, injecting local anesthetics with epinephrine is advisable. However, hypersensitivity to anesthetic drugs as well as the reaction toward the epinephrine (arrhythmias, etc.) should be considered.

7.2 External Auditory Meatus: Skin Lacerations and Exostoses

The type of incision depends on the surgeon. Either making the incision endaurally may expose the surgical field to more interactions, the incision itself is not a matter of increased risk of complication. There may be delayed epithelization over the porus of the external auditory canal (EAC).

If there are exostoses of the EAC, one should consider whether to do stage operation or not. Multiple lacerations of skin flap will increase the risk of infection and delayed healing of the surgical wound. Small exostoses will not pose any problem.

Additionally, there may be laceration of the skin flap. As long as there appears no tissue loss

---

Electronic supplementary material The online version of this chapter (doi:10.1007/978-3-319-28576-4_7) contains supplementary material, which is available to authorized users.

O.N. Ozgirgin
Sogutozu Otolaryngology Department, Bayindir Hospital, Ankara, Turkey
e-mail: ozgirgin@politzersociety.org

I. Sziklai (ed.), *Surgery of Stapes Fixations*, DOI 10.1007/978-3-319-28576-4_7

(i.e., the skin flap may be torn around the shaft of the drill which may result with loss of the skin tissue) the healing process will be good. If there is a simple laceration, putting the edges of the skin flap will serve for perfect epithelization. If there is tissue loss, the EAC bone should not be left uncovered and temporalis muscle fascia will be a very good material to cover the bone to be inserted under the skin flaps.

It is well known that the skin close to the annulus of the tympanic membrane (TM) is much thinner and easier to be ruptured. So much attention is needed while elevating the part of the skin medial to the EAM.

7.3 Tympanic Membrane: Laceration

When reached to the annulus of TM, sharper dissectors need to be used to keep the integrity of the fibrous annulus and the tympanic membrane. The most convenient part to access the middle ear is the Rivinus notch. This will help preserve the annulus and the tympanic membrane. Principally, the meatal skin and the annulus should be elevated between the two sutures, tympanosquamosa and tympanomastoid. The angle of approach between these two structures will expose the two window areas as well as the malleus. If exposure of the anterior malleolar ligament is necessary in case of malleus fixation, anterior elevation will be needed.

In any case, extreme care should be taken to keep the TM intact. In case of laceration, the TM perforation should be repaired meticulously. Either temporal muscle fascia or tragal cartilage perichondrium will serve as a good material to repair (Video 7.1). And during the early postoperative period, it is necessary to be sure about the complete epithelization over the TM. TM perforations exposing the middle ear to infections will create the risk of otitis media and labyrinthitis that will result in sensorineural hearing loss.

The chordal crest will frequently prevent the exposure and access to the incudostapedial complex and will need to be removed. The instruments to remove the crest are the microdrill and bone curettes. This depends on the practice of the surgeon. While doing this, one should keep in mind the distance between the crest and the facial recess. Here is the stage of the surgery where the facial nerve comes into the risk of damage. The drill and the curette should always be under vision, and they should never be inserted over the facial recess.

7.4 Chorda Tympani

There is another formation that is more prone to injury during the exposure of the incudostapedial complex, and that is the chorda tympani. The chorda is situated just beneath the crest, and it is very easy to damage the nerve. Accessing the middle ear through the Rivinus notch will also serve for keeping the nerve safe. But still the position of the nerve will mask the incudomalleolar joint to go through. In most cases, elevating the chorda tympani anterior will be needed, and this will give a tension to the nerve, making the patient suffer from taste disturbances following the surgery.

Until recently, there has been a discussion of cutting the chorda tympani instead of keeping intact but stretching. And the authors favoring to cut the nerve argued that the taste disturbance would be much less and short term [3].

The sensation for taste is also supplied by the glossopharyngeal nerve and circumvallate papillae on the posterior tongue. Even the palate is supplied by greater superficial petrosal nerve and the throat by vagus, and they serve for taste sensation. There may be cross-innervation from the contralateral chorda tympani nerve. Unilateral damage affects the whole-mouth taste perception slightly [4].

However, another study conducted by Miuchi et al. [5] shows that the electrogustometry thresholds kept their high values for a year or longer among the patients who suffered from taste problems following the stapes surgery.

The author suggests to keep the nerve intact thinner which is the sign of losing some fibers of it.

7.5 Incudostapedial Joint: Dislocation

It is necessary to expose the long process of incus, pyramidal eminence, and the stapedius tendon for a full access to the oval window. Within the standard steps of the surgery, it is essential to check the mobility of malleus to discard the possibility of its fixation. Afterwards, the surgical approach for the replacement of stapes with the piston prosthesis will come. Here, the order of interventions may differ due to the surgeon. Some keep the incudostapedial joint untouched until the insertion of piston prosthesis is performed.

The author's approach is detaching the incudostapedial joint, cutting the stapedius tendon, cutting the crura to remove the superstructure of the stapes, opening the stapedotomy hole by using laser to the footplate, and then inserting the piston prosthesis. This is the procedure that is accomplished mostly by laser users.

Removing the incudostapedial joint is a mechanical process. One should take extreme care not to dislocate the incus during detaching the joint. The position of the incus is also under stress while working over the oval window and footplate. During inserting the instruments and taking them out, one can dislocate the incus. In case of its dislocation, there will be some methods to remedy this. If the incus is completely dislocated, it will be necessary to use the malleus to vestibule piston prosthesis, to make malleostapedotomy (Video 7.2). There are several prostheses designed for this purpose. Some of them are designed to fit exactly in the left or right ear. It is necessary to keep both piston prostheses for right and left ready to be used in case needed. Some prostheses are versatile and can be used in both sides.

The author's choice is using the Fisch titanium prosthesis for malleostapedotomy cases. The shaft of the piston is shorter, but the neck of the piston can be bent to give the angle to bridge the malleus to the oval window. It is necessary to attach the hook of the piston prosthesis as much closer to the processus brevis of the malleus to make it stable and secure. This will also help the tympanic membrane to cover the hook of the prosthesis better.

If the incus is dislocated but still in contact with the malleus, it may be better to stage the operation and leave the stapedectomy to a second stage which may be 3–6 months later. The time will serve for rebuilding the contact between the two ossicles, malleus, and incus to vibrate as a unique formation. The second stage will be much more effective in conducting the vibrations from TM to vestibule with the inserted piston prosthesis.

A case of incudostapedial dislocation that has been repaired by "fibrin glue" is reported [6]. The technique has been reported as safe, rapid, and accurate. And the use of fibrin glue was also favored by the audiometric results.

In a standard procedure, the incudostapedial joint is detached, the stapedius tendon is cut, and the stapes superstructure is removed. This can be accomplished by using several instruments. Crura scissors may be used to cut the crura, or they may be broken by pulling and pushing the crura anteroposteriorly. This kind of procedure will create mechanical stress to the footplate, and in some instances, the whole stapes may come out that will result in total stapedectomy. The surgeon should get ready for such a complication, and in such condition the oval window has to be sealed with perichondrium to prevent perilymph fistula formation.

If lasers are being used, the posterior crus is evaporated, but in most instances, the position of the stapes does not permit access to the anterior crus. However, the anterior crus is much thinner than the posterior, and as long as the posterior crus is completely cut, the anterior crus will be easily broken without creating any mechanical stress to the footplate. Wegner et al. [7] in their systematic review on comparing conventional techniques with laser found no evidence that either the laser fenestration or conventional fenestration technique is superior to each other, but they also stressed that there could be increased risk of footplate fracture and SNHL when micro-instruments or micro-drills are used. Fang et al. [8] also support the micro-traumatic effect of lasers as compared with the conventional

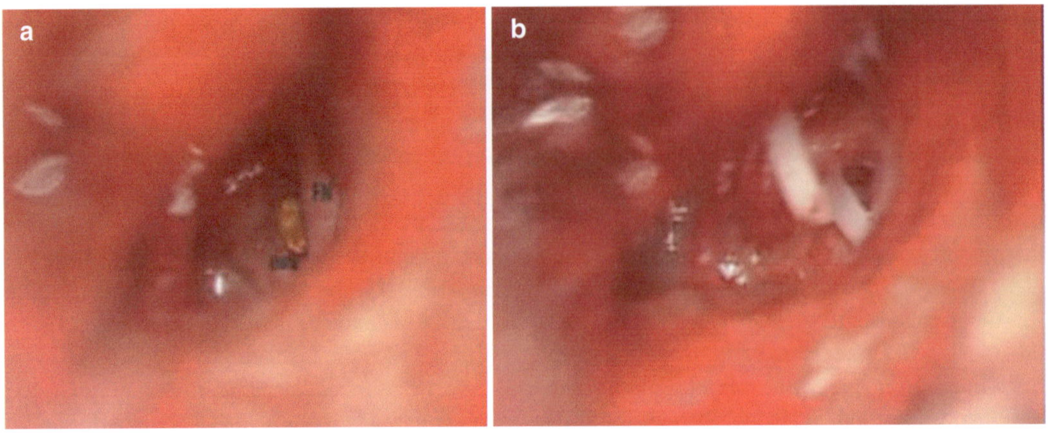

Fig. 7.1 (**a**, **b**) Anteriorly located facial nerve permitting insertion of 0.4 mm piston prosthesis. *FN* facial nerve, *OWN* oval window

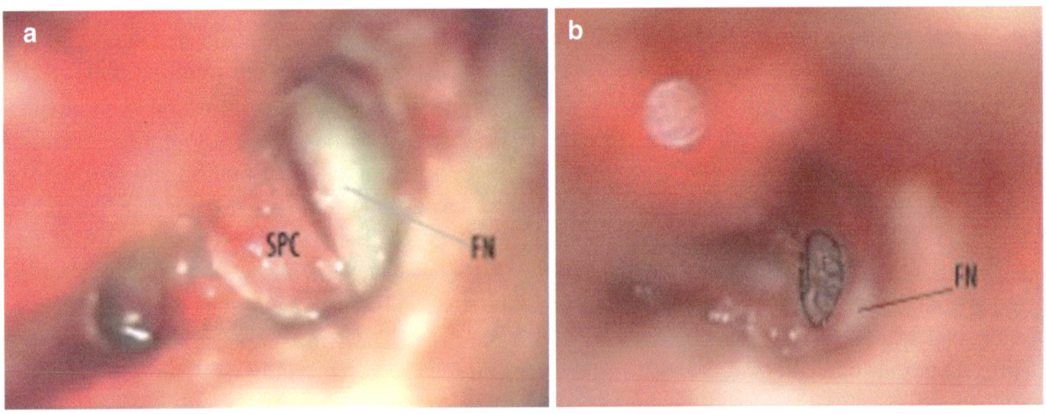

Fig. 7.2 (**a**) Protruding facial nerve and stapes crura that do not allow intervention over the oval window. (**b**) Facial nerve partially closing the oval window. *FN* facial nerve, *SPC* stapes crura

instruments, concluding with the favor of using lasers in stapedotomy surgery.

7.6 Facial Nerve Abnormalities

The facial nerve plays a dominant role in this part of the surgery. Mostly, its position allows the surgeon to access the footplate and perform the procedure on it. But the condition is not the same in every case.

The facial nerve may be displaced anteriorly to mask the footplate, the fallopian canal may be dehiscent, and the nerve itself may be exposed completely, and it may even be enlarged to cover the whole window and the stapes footplate. There may be even a neurinoma formation of the facial nerve in proximity to the stapes (Figs. 7.1,7.2, and 7.3; Videos 7.3 and 7.4).

For an experienced surgeon, it is very difficult to damage the nerve as long as it is under vision. The challenge is how much to retract the nerve or how much to drill the anterior niche of the oval window for creating the stapedotomy hole.

The condition here is, how much the nerve is to be retracted, to allow the piston prosthesis being inserted. Neff et al. [9] suggest using the Robinson prosthesis and inserting as it indents the facial nerve when significant prolapse of the facial nerve is present. Another question to be responded is whether the permanent contact of

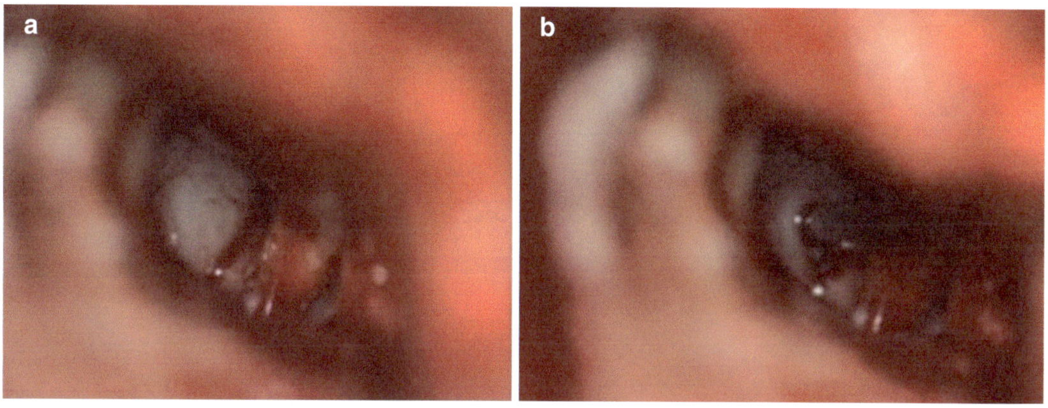

Fig. 7.3 (**a**, **b**) Facial neurinoma replacing all the space toward the crura

the nerve with the piston prosthesis could trigger the neurinoma formation.

The safe distance to be drilled anteriorly is less than a millimeter; otherwise the basal turn of the cochlea can be damaged. Another question is how much feasible is drilling or removing the bone over the fallopian canal nearby the oval window to retract the facial nerve. Leaving the surgery will be the best option in such threatening conditions.

7.7 The Footplate

Most of the annoying complications are related with the footplate. This is because the complication related with the footplate and the vestibule almost results in sensorineural hearing loss. It is not a good feeling either for the patient or for the surgeon when a hearing restoration surgery results in total hearing loss.

There are several factors that can cause unfavorable result. The footplate can be fragile (biscuit type) and can be obliterative, the fixation may not be total, and the distance between the footplate and the saccule may be inconsistent. To make the surgery safer, there are surgeons who keep the stapes intact until the prosthesis is inserted.

The lasers have been introduced into the stapes surgery to refrain applying mechanical pressure over the footplate and to make precise opening for insertion of the piston prosthesis.

Besides their safety in regard to the footplate manipulations, their success on reducing the air–bone gaps was discussed by many articles already published. A meta-analysis conducted by Fang et al. [8] pointed out that there was significant difference between the laser and non-laser groups in the closure of air–bone gap.

Regard to the safety of lasers in stapes surgery, Matkovic et al. [10] mentioned the advantages as avoiding any trauma to the membranous labyrinth and also simplifying and shortening the procedure. Motta and Moscillo [11] noted that by using lasers it would be easier to make the edge of the opening smooth and even adjust the diameter of fenestra to the prosthesis caliber.

If the footplate is thick and the otospongiosis is obliterative, it is easier to go through by using micro-drills. Micro drills are fine for this purpose. Reversely using lasers for obliterative otosclerosis will cause accumulation of heat that will also increase the temperature in the vestibule. So to reduce side effects of the heat, the laser should be applied with intervals and additionally the charcoal should be removed in layers.

Malafronte et al. [12] made a classification of footplate for the cases of otosclerosis that could be helpful for reminding the surgeon in terms of intraoperative complications. The authors suggest three different forms of footplate in otosclerosis: blue otosclerosis, white otosclerosis, and obliterative otosclerosis. The blue footplate is composed of healthy and elastic bone resistant to the trauma due to the superstructure removal and the fenestration. In white otosclerosis, the otosclerotic focus involves most of the footplate,

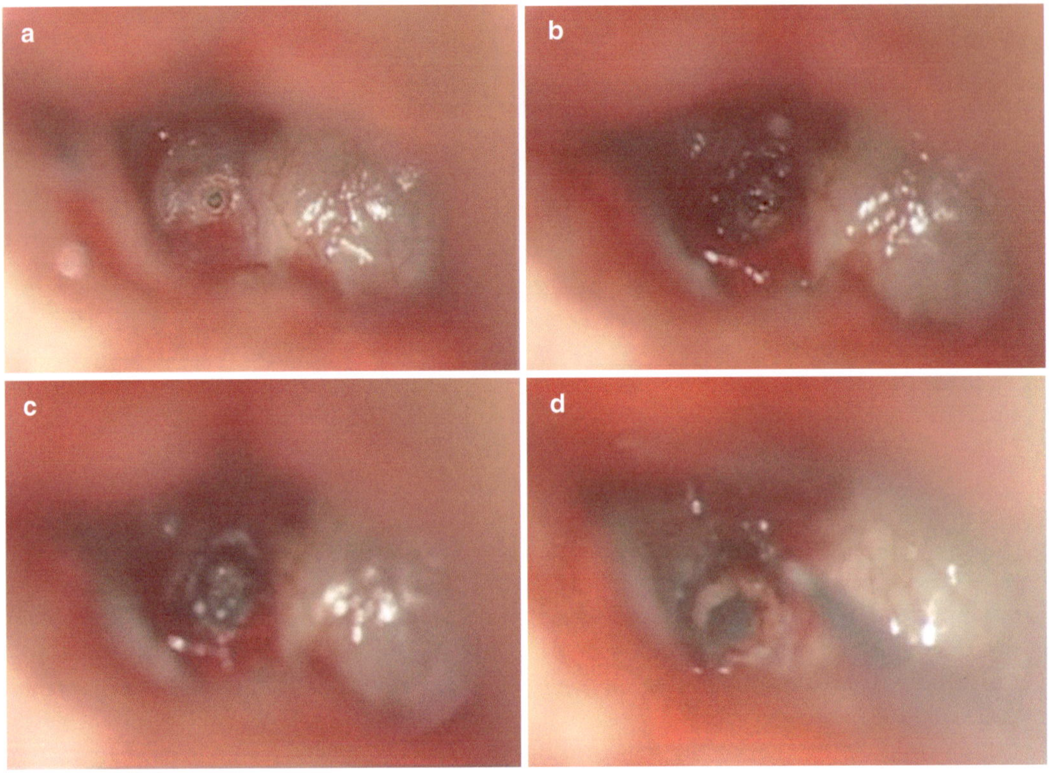

Fig. 7.4 (**a–d**) Obliterative otosclerosis. Using laser and needles for removing the sclerotic tissue in layers for a safe opening to the vestibule

which becomes fragile, vitreous, and less resistant to trauma due to surgical manipulations. When the otosclerotic foci involve only the footplate, it is also called as biscuit otosclerosis. The biscuit footplate is the most susceptible one to complications such as floating footplate. This type (biscuit) confines to 22.8 % of cases. In obliterative otosclerosis, the footplate is invisible (Fig. 7.4a–d; Video 7.5).

Further, the authors [13] also suggested using CO2 laser especially in white otosclerosis cases which could significantly reduce the intraoperative complications.

The two mostly used lasers in stapes surgery are argon and CO2. The properties of these two lasers are completely different. Argon is similar to KTP and their wavelengths are 488 and 532 nm, respectively. The beams of these two lasers are visible but are not absorbed by water. This means that the laser beam can access to the inner ear membranes, so there is a potential of injury on the saccule or utricle when directly applied toward the vestibule.

CO2 laser has wavelength 10,600 nm. Excess energy created by CO2 laser is highly absorbed by the perilymph and because of this reason is safer than argon and KTP in terms of their effects to the inner ear. However, the laser beams are not visible so they cannot be delivered by silica fibers. When used through an operating microscope via a micromanipulator, the beams have to be coupled with an aiming beam (helium–neon laser) for clinical use. So until recently one-shot CO2 laser stapedotomy was performed to achieve 0.5–0.7 mm in diameter hole nearly round, with clean-cut edges. Recently, a handheld delivery system has been manufactured to overcome the aiming beam problems such as potential risks of incorrect aiming and laser beam misalignment. In addition, there is the possibility for the surgeon to use the laser with a handheld device just as it is for argon laser. Vincent et al. [14] suggest that

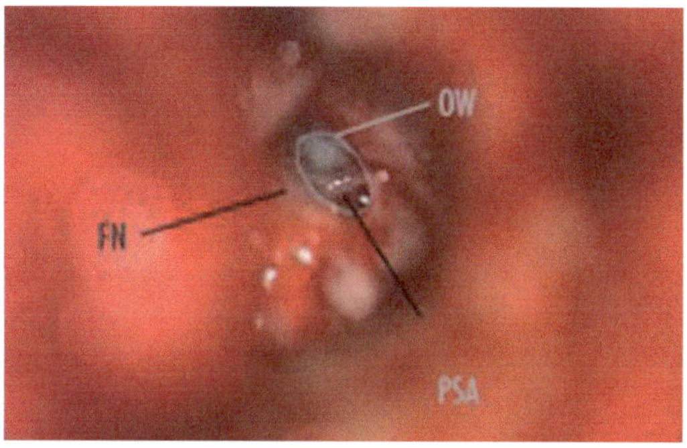

Fig. 7.5 Persistent stapedial artery crossing the oval window. *FN* facial nerve, *OW* oval window, *PSA* persistent stapedial artery

their study confirm the usefulness of both lasers, argon and CO2 laser, and add that they had a case of sensorineural hearing loss with argon where no problems existed with fiber CO2 laser.

Sometimes the stapedial artery still persists as it is crossing across the footplate (Video 7.6). The bleeding through it will be troublesome. It may be coagulated if it is not too large, but one should keep in mind the possibility of combination of aberrant internal carotid artery and persistent stapedial artery [15]. During embyonal development, meningeal artery is formed through a branch of stapedial artery. Anastomoses develop between the ventral branches and the external carotid artery. The stapedial artery normally degenerates by gestational week 10, separating the internal carotid artery from the external carotid artery. However, persistence of the stapedial artery into postnatal life may indicate the anastomoses between the internal and external carotid arteries can occur [16] (Fig. 7.5).

7.8 The Vestibule

Preoperative high-resolution computed tomography of the ear will be very helpful on understanding the state of the oval window and the type of the lesion affecting it. So the surgeon will have opinion about what kind of difficulty is waiting for him, and of course this will be the opportunity to inform the patient preoperatively. Purohit et al. [17] list the reporting points in CTs for stapes surgery as size and location of plaques, status of oval and round windows, facial nerve canal, concurrent middle ear pathologies, ossicular chain integrity, sinus plate and jugular bulb, inner ear pathology, and the opposite ear. The aqueducts of cochlea and the vestibule should be included in this list (Fig. 7.6).

The footplate may be mobilized during the surgery. When this occurs, if mechanical procedures are being used with micro-pick opening or micro-drill applications, it will be easy to push the footplate toward the vestibule. When the annual ligament of the footplate corrupts, the footplate falls down the vestibule. This is something very challenging. Leaving the bony footplate in the vestibule will create vestibular symptoms seriously that will never be tolerated by the patient. Reversely fishing the footplate from the vestibule will result in the rupture of the vestibular membranes (saccule and/or utricle) which will result in total hearing loss.

There are some measures described to perform in such a situation.

Dropping some blood to clot in the vestibule can help to remove the footplate by suctioning the clot without giving any harm to the membranous labyrinth and even not aspirating the perilymph. This is logical but I am not sure how effectively it works.

If the footplate in the vestibule is under vision, drilling nearby the niche of the oval window to extract it with a fine 90° pick can help solving the problem.

Another precaution is keeping the mucosa of the promontorium in continuum with the footplate intact. In case of broken part of footplate, the mucosa attached to it will keep it from falling into the vestibule, and even leaving it hanging nearby the footplate opening will not cause any problem. This is the condition that occurs in practice and helps the surgery being safe.

When using lasers, charcoal appears over the footplate and sometimes the fragments of the charcoal fall down the vestibule. This never causes a problem. Even if small fragments of bone of the footplate fall down, the only symptom will be the temporary positional vertigo.

A case of intraoperative loss of a piston prosthesis into the vestibule has been reported. In this case, while attempting to correct the wire angulation, the piston disrupted free from the wire and

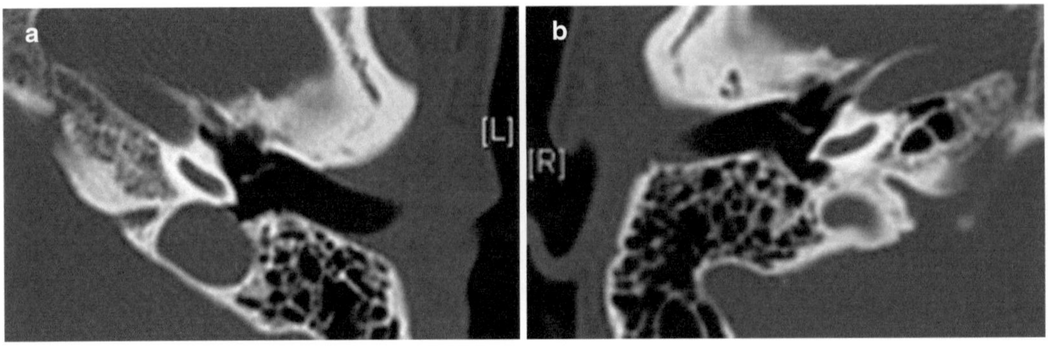

Fig. 7.6 (**a**, **b**) Cochlear aqueduct as observed in axial sections of computed tomographies

sank into the vestibule out of sight. Even if the authors decided to leave the prosthesis within the vestibule, the patient did not show a sensorineural hearing loss nor vertigo [18].

7.9 Suctioning Through the Stapedotomy Opening

When working over the footplate, one of the precautions that one should consider is not to suction the perilymph. The direct aspiration through the opening over the footplate will create negative pressure all over the labyrinth and will cause the collapse and the rupture of the membranes, which results in total hearing loss. The tip of the suction tube should always in distant to the vestibular opening.

Ikeda et al. [19] measured the endolymphatic potential among the guinea pigs grouped as without suctioning, indirect suctioning, and direct suctioning through the oval window. They concluded that even gentle suctioning and removal of the vestibular perilymph can cause a mild decrease in EP even without damaging the inner ear structures.

7.10 Oozing and Gusher

One of the most unfavorable complications of stapes surgery is the perilymph leak with pressure. One should not mix oozing with the gusher. Oozing is the pressure over the perilymphatic compartment that causes the continuous flow of the perilymph toward the middle ear following stapedotomy. However, this will decrease and stop within a while. Inserting perichondrium beneath the piston prosthesis or fascia or packing around the piston will successfully treat the condition without further perilymph leak. Reversely, the gusher is the spurt out of the perilymph. Even by waiting, the pressure will not decrease. The gusher is also known as the leak of cerebrospinal fluid and thought to be due to the direct connection between the perilymphatic space and the CSF. Either the cochleariform aqueduct [20] or vestibular aqueduct can serve for this if enlarged and also in cases with a defect in the fundus of the internal auditory meatus. This is one of the reasons why high-resolution computed tomography is needed before the surgery (Fig. 7.6).

Fortunately, this is a rare condition. Causse [21] estimasted an 0.03 % incidence rate. The real gusher mostly appears in congenital stapes fixation.

There are still few things to manage the condition. Hyperventilation of the patient will decrease the CSF pressure and will help the condition to be managed. Repositioning the patient to reverse Trendelenburg position may be helpful. Additionally, CSF drainage by inserting a lumbar paravertebral catheter will be very effective even during the surgery. During the surgery, there are also some measures to be taken. The first is to pack efficiently the oval window to stop the flow and leave the surgery. This will serve for keeping the bone conduction hearing levels in place to allow patient using hearing aid. Another issue is to completely seal the stapedotomy opening and inserting the prosthesis also to make some

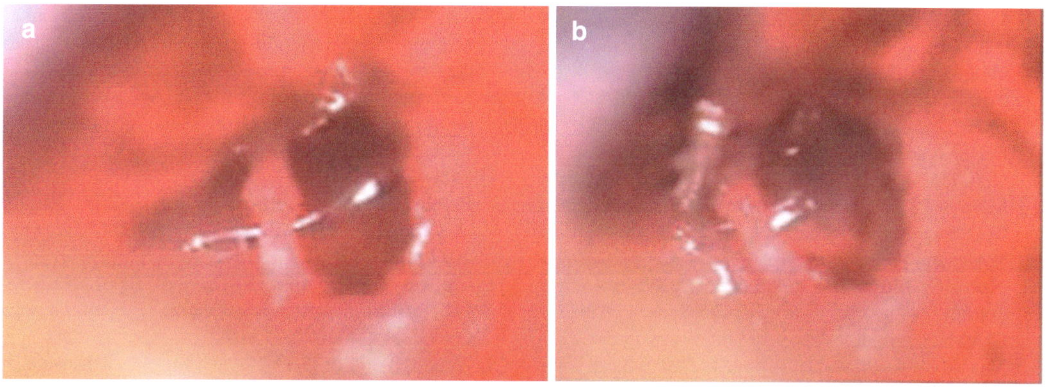

Fig. 7.7 CSF filling the middle ear following the first shot of argon laser

pressure over the graft to help total sealing. Following the surgery, prescribing diuretics will keep the pressure low. Additionally, the patient should keep his/her head elevated. There may be cases in which the perilymph/CSF can wet the dressing (Fig. 7.7a–b).

Causse et al. [22] defined two clues that should call the attention of the surgeon to the possibility of gusher: an avascular congenital middle ear and abnormally anterior insertion of the posterior crus of the footplate.

The perilymph gusher when manifested causes sensorineural hearing loss in more than 50 % of the patients.

When using the hand drills or picks during the stapedotomy, the surgeon should take care not to insert the instrument toward the vestibule; otherwise the saccule can be ruptured which will result in sensorineural hearing loss.

Even with the lasers, it is very important for the surgeon to know the potential hazards of the tool being used. In this instance, the type of laser becomes so important. If laser is needed to be used following opening the footplate, beams should be absorbed by the fluid so that it would not injure the membranes of the labyrinth which would result in sensorineural hearing loss. Penetration by the laser is not the only risk but also elevation of the temperature within the vestibule will threat the neuroepithelium.

Carbon dioxide laser is very convenient in such cases, as the beams of argon laser will not be absorbed by the fluid (perilymph) and will go through the vestibule.

Conclusion

The surgery for otosclerosis is a refined approach to replace immobilized stapes with piston prosthesis. Whatever the technique and device used, the surgeon should take care about the stapes footplate and the vestibule to be more precise to achieve better hearing and to avoid revision surgery (Videos 7.7 and 7.8).

References

1. Schuknecht HF. Sensorineural hearing loss following stapedectomy. Acta Otolaryngol. 1962;54:336–48. Guyot JP, Sakbeni K. Patients' lives following stapedectomy complications. Adv Otorhinolaryngol. 2007;65:348–52.
2. Guyot JP, Sakbeni K. Patients' lives following stapedectomy complications. Adv Otorhinolaryngol. 2007;65:348–52.
3. Gopalan P, Kumar M, Gupta D, Phillipps JJ. A study of chorda tympani nerve injury and related symptoms following middle-ear surgery. J Laryngol Otol. 2005;119:189–92.
4. Clark MPA, O'Malley S. Chorda tympani nerve function after middle ear surgery. Otol Neurotol. 2007;28: 335–40.
5. Miuchi S, Sakagami M, Tsuzuki K, Noguchi K, Mishiro Y, Katsura H. Taste disturbance after stapes surgery – clinical and experimental study. Acta Otolaryngol Suppl. 2009;562:71–8.
6. Nikolaidis V. Traumatic dislocation of the incudostapedial joint repaired with fibrin tissue adhesive. Laryngoscope. 2011;121:577–9.
7. Wegner I, Kamalski D, Tange RA, Vincent R, Stegeman I, van der Heijden GJM, Grolman W. Laser versus conventional fenestration in stapedotomy for otosclerosis: a systematic review Laryngoscope, 2013;124:1687–93, 2014.

8. Fang L, Lin H, Zhang TY, Tan J. Laser versus non-laser stapedotomy in otosclerosis: a systematic review and meta-analysis. Auris Nasus Larynx. 2014;41:337–42.
9. Neff BA, Lippy WH, Schuring AG, Rizer FM. Stapedectomy in patients with a prolapsed facial nerve. Otolaryngol Head Neck Surg. 2004;130: 597–603.
10. Matkovic S, Kitanoski B, Malicevic Z. Advantages of CO2 laser use in surgical management of otosclerosis. Vojnosanit Pregl. 2003;60:273–8.
11. Motta G, Moscillo L. Functional results in stapedotomy with and without CO(2)laser. ORL J Otorhinolaryngol Relat Spec. 2002;64:307–10.
12. Malafronte G, Filosa B, Cantone E. New macroscopic classification of stapedio-ovalar otosclerosis: a simplified rating for training in stapedotomy. Otol Neurotol. 2008;29:889–92.
13. Malafronte G, Filosa B, Barillari MR. Stapedotomy: is the color of the footplate important in the choice of the type of perforator? Otol Neurotol. 2011;32: 1047–149.
14. Vincent R, Bittermann AJN, Oates J, Sperling N, Grolman W. KTP Versus CO2 laser fiber stapedotomy for primary otosclerosis: results of a new comparative series with the otology-neurotology database. Otol Neurotol. 2012;33:928–33.
15. Lau CC, Oghalai JS, Jackler RK. Combination of aberrant internal carotid artery and persistent stapedial artery. Otol Neurotol. 2004;25:850–1.
16. Lasjaunias P, Santoyo-Vazquez A. Segmental agenesis of the internal carotid artery: angiographic aspects with embryological discussion. Anat Clin. 1984;6: 133–41.
17. Purohit B, Hermans R, Op de beeck K. Imaging in otosclerosis: a pictorial review. Insights Imaging. 2014;5:245–52.
18. Carlson ML, Haberman RS. Loss of stapes prosthesis into vestibule during stapedectomy: a case report. Otol Neurotol. 2007;28:510–2.
19. Ikeda R, Nakaya K, Oshima H, Oshima T, Kawase T, Kobayashi T. Effect of aspiration of perilymph during stapes surgery on the endocochlear potential of guinea pig. Otolaryngol Head Neck Surg. 2011;145(5): 801–5.
20. Farrior B, Endicott JN. Congenital mixed deafness: cerebrospinal fluid otorrhea. Ablation of the aqueduct of the cochlea. Laryngoscope. 1971;81:684–99.
21. Causse J, Causse JB. Eighteen-year report on stapedectomy. I: problems of stapedial fixation. Clin Otolaryngol. 1980;5:49–59.
22. Causse JB, Causse JR, Wiet RJ, Yoo TJ. Complications of stapedectomies. Am J Otol. 1983;4:275–80.

8 Transcanal Endoscopic Stapedotomy

Lela Migirov

8.1 Introduction

Endoscopes have rapidly become widely accepted in the performance of ear surgery. The indications for minimally invasive endoscopic and endoscope-assisted surgical techniques extended from cases of cholesteatoma to various ear pathologies and include myringoplasty, stapes surgery, cochlear implantation, and inner ear surgery. My personal experience with more than 200 transcanal endoscopic surgeries demonstrated the superiority of the endoscopic view of the middle ear (ME) structures compared to a microscopic view, the latter being defined and limited by the narrowest segment of the ear canal [18, 19]. Stapedotomy can be technically difficult and challenging due to anatomic variations in size, configuration, shape, or irregularity of the external ear canal. The stapes and oval window niche (OWN) can be obscured by the scutum. Good exposure of the OWN allowing a fenestration of the footplate and clipping of the prosthesis onto the incus can be obtained by reclining (pushing apart or stretching) the chorda tympani nerve (CTN) in most stapes surgeries performed using the microscope. When the posterior part of the bony annulus is removed to visualize the stapes, the CTN can be occasionally touched and stretched [20]. Excessive removal of the bone for better visualization of the ME structures can result not only in damage to the CTN but also in subluxation of the incus [8, 13, 15]. The rate of postoperative taste disorders or tongue symptoms after stapes surgery is high (20–60 %) in patients whose CTN was only manipulated and in patients whose CTN was transected, and many authors recommend appropriate preoperative counseling despite the transient nature of symptoms in some cases [4, 9, 17, 20, 25, 28]. Endoscope-assisted stapedotomy was first described by Poe [23]; however the data on the fully endoscopic stapedotomy is very limited [12, 19, 21, 26]. The surgeons performing transcanal endoscopic stapedotomy (TES) showed that an endoscopic approach to the ME obviates the need to divide the CTN in order to obtain adequate access to the stapes and OWN [12, 19, 21, 26]. The CTN may not be exposed at all during a transcanal endoscopic procedure, while it is near always at risk and must occasionally be sacrificed in patients who are operated under a conventional otomicroscope.

I have started TES with an intent to simplify the surgical procedure for otosclerosis and prove the possibility of avoiding injury to the CTN when attempting to achieve visibility of the ME structures.

L. Migirov, MD
Department of Otolaryngology Head and Neck Surgery, Sheba Medical Center, Sackler School of Medicine, Tel Aviv University, Tel Hashomer, Ramat Gan 52621, Israel
e-mail: migirovl@gmail.com

I. Sziklai (ed.), *Surgery of Stapes Fixations*, DOI 10.1007/978-3-319-28576-4_8

8.2 Surgical Technique

The external ear canal was injected with lidocaine 1 % with 1:100,000 epinephrine. The position of the patients was the same as for routine otomicroscopic ear surgeries. A fully endoscopic transcanal procedure was undertaken using rigid endoscopes 3-mm diameter, 14-cm length, 0° and 30°. Angled picks, curved micro aspirators, curved scissors, and forceps were used in addition to the routine otologic micro-instruments. A posterior tympanomeatal flap was elevated transmeatally with the 0° endoscope and then transposed anteriorly (Fig. 8.1). Cotton balls soaked in 1:2000 were placed in the ear canal for a few minutes in case of excessive bleeding during tympanomeatal flap elevation. Stapes fixation was confirmed by gentle testing of ossicular chain mobility (Figs. 8.2 and 8.3). The stapes tendon was cut with curved microscissors, and the stapes was separated from the incus in the incudostapedial joint (Fig. 8.4). The anterior and posterior stapedial crura were carefully fractured, and the superstructure was removed (Figs. 8.5 and 8.6). The distance between the footplate and medial surface of the long process of the incus was measured to determine the required prosthesis size (Figs. 8.7 and 8.8). The hole in the footplate was created with a Skeeter microdrill using a 0.5-mm diameter diamond burr or gentle perforator (Fig. 8.9). A platinum/fluoroplastic piston prosthesis (0.4-mm diameter, 4.5/4.75-mm length) was placed into this hole and fitted along the long process of the incus (Figs. 8.10 and 8.11).

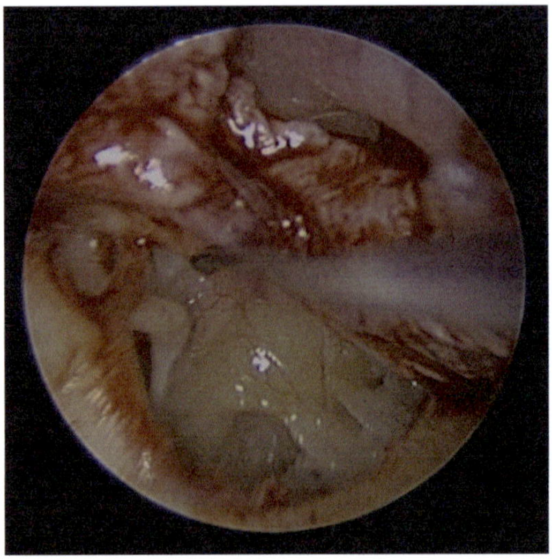

Fig. 8.2 Endoscopic view of the right middle ear after an elevation of the tympanomeatal flap: good access to the stapes and to the oval window niche was achieved without removal of the scutum and without touching the chorda tympani nerve. Touching the malleus for examination of its movement

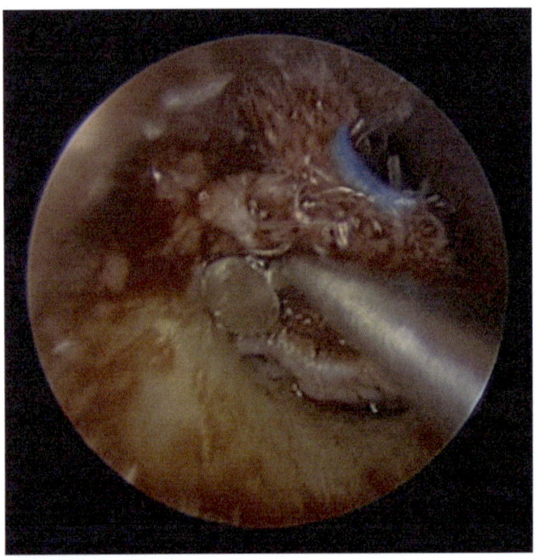

Fig. 8.1 Endoscopic view of the right middle ear: elevation of the tympanomeatal flap

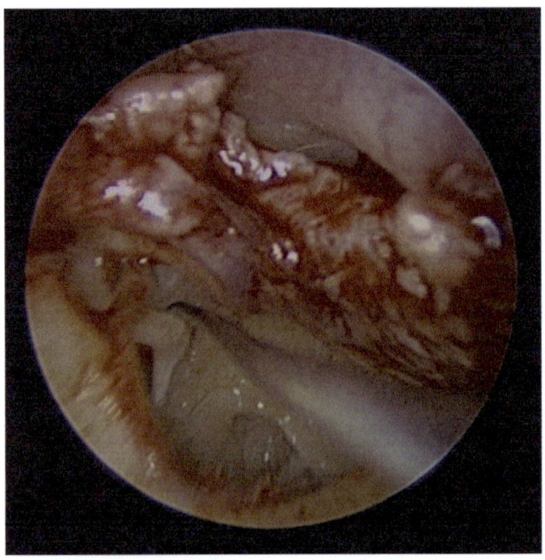

Fig. 8.3 Endoscopic view of the right middle ear: examination of incudal movement

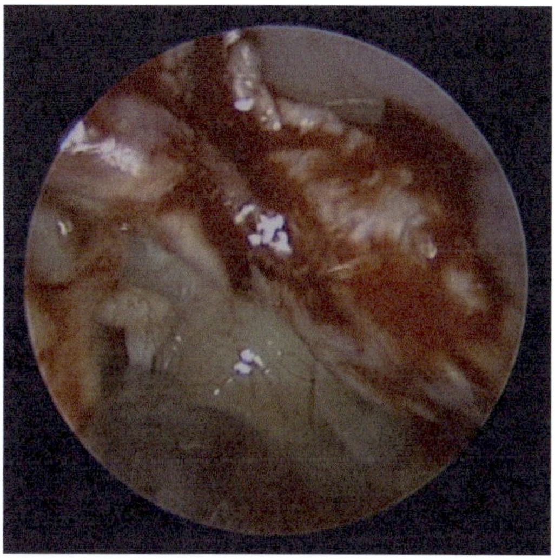

Fig. 8.4 Endoscopic view of the right ear: cutting of the stapedius

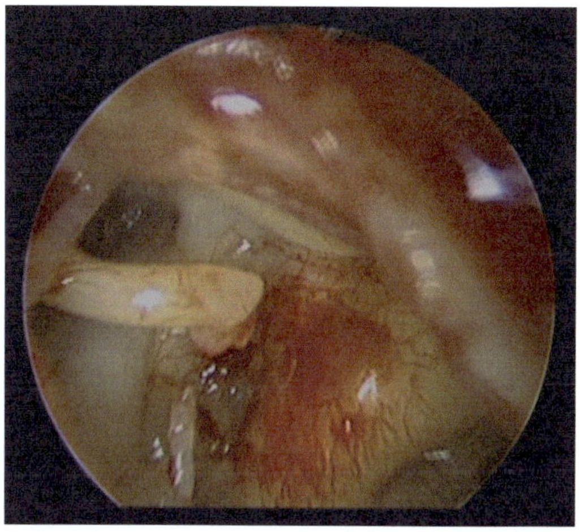

Fig. 8.6 Endoscopic view of the right ear: focus on the stapedius, incudostapedial joint, stapes, oval window niche, and facial nerve

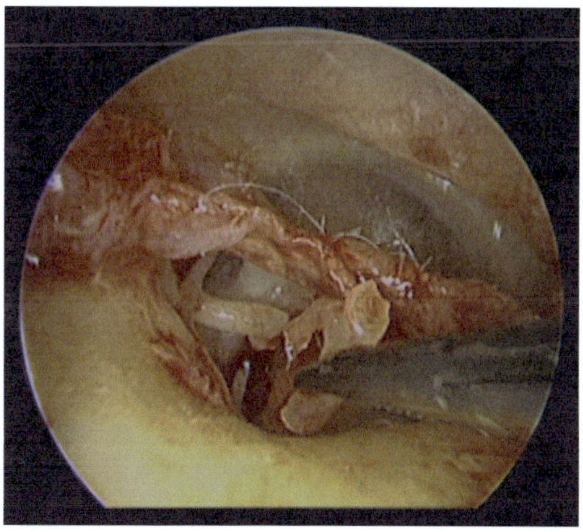

Fig. 8.5 Endoscopic view of the right ear: removal of stapes

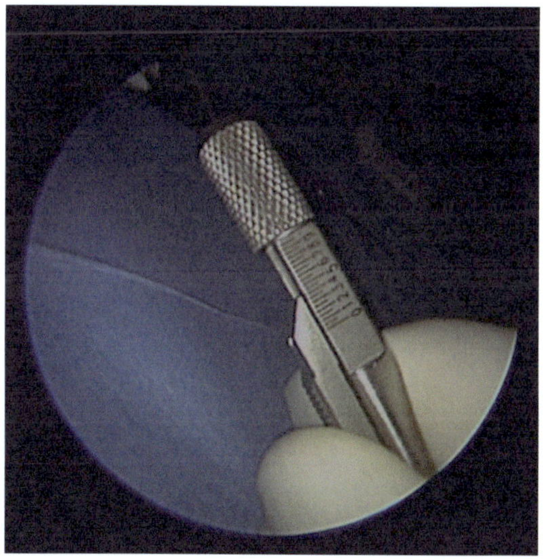

Fig. 8.7 Endoscopic view of the measuring tool

The appropriate ossicular chain movement with the replaced stapes was ensured by malleus palpation. A small piece of fat has been taken from the posterior surface of lobule and placed surrounding the prosthesis. The tympanomeatal flap was repositioned, and the external auditory canal was filled with Gelfoam® soaked in eardrops containing antibiotics. Frequent suctioning was avoided in any stage of surgery, especially after fenestration.

Fifteen females and four males (age range 23–74 years, mean 45.7 years) diagnosed as having otosclerosis underwent TES (without conversion to a conventional otomicroscopic technique) by the author between April 2012 and December 2013. One patient underwent bilateral sequential TES with a 12-month gap between the surgeries. Overall, 11 right ears and nine left ears were operated. Eleven procedures were performed

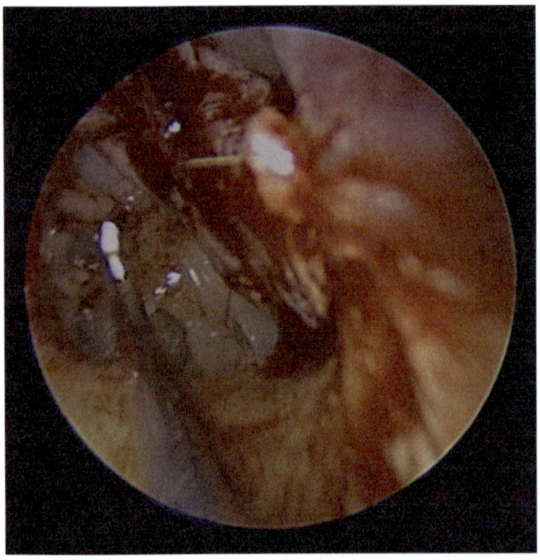

Fig. 8.8 Endoscopic view of the right ear: measure the distance between the oval window niche and incus

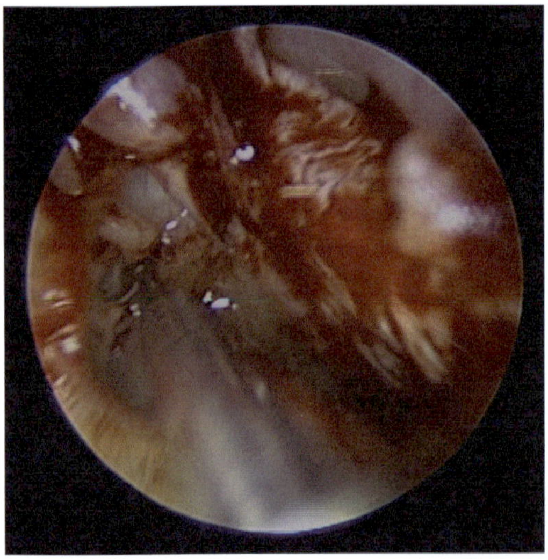

Fig. 8.9 Endoscopic view of the right ear: fenestration with a Skeeter drill

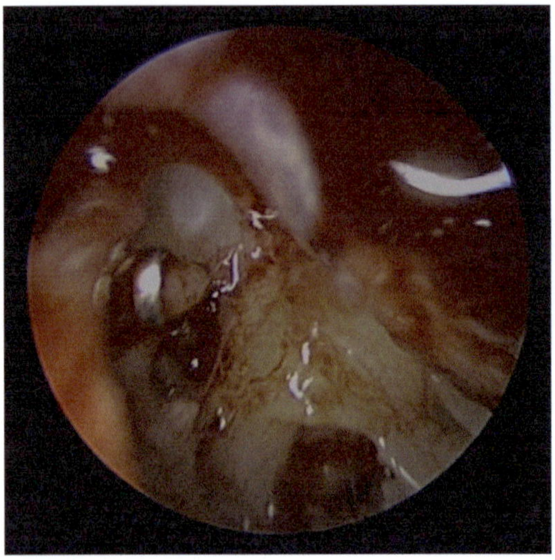

Fig. 8.10 Endoscopic view of the right ear: after the placement of prosthesis

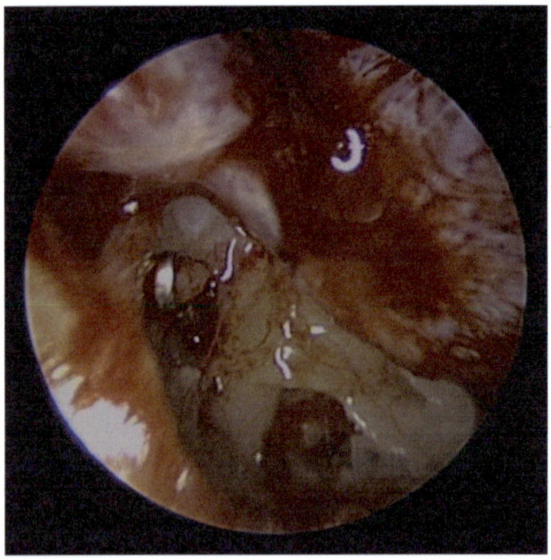

Fig. 8.11 Endoscopic overview of the right ear after the transcanal endoscopic stapedotomy

under general anesthesia, and the other nine surgeries were carried out under local anesthesia. All the surgeries were performed with a 0° endoscope, while a 30° endoscope was required to better visualize the OWN, the anterior crus of the stapes, the tympanic portion of the facial nerve, and the pyramidal eminence in seven cases due to bony overhang in the posterior tympanum. Endoscopic view of the ME was sufficient in all cases and does not require any curettage or drilling of the scutum or mobilization of the CTN (Figs. 8.1, 8.2, 8.3, 8.4, 8.5, 8.6, 8.8, 8.9, 8.10, and 8.11). Four patients had narrow footplate with dehiscent facial nerve-covered footplate partially in two of them. Overall, facial was dehiscent in its tympanic portion in 6/20 (30 %) cases. Two patients had an obliterated footplate. A 4.5-mm prosthesis was used in 17 cases and a

4.75-mm prosthesis in three. One patient developed vertigo 30 h post-stapedotomy and was treated with intravenous amoxicillin-clavulanate and steroids. Those symptoms resolved 1 week following surgery. There was no need in removal of the scutum in presented series. However, some surgeons utilize curetting or drilling of bone overhang despite the use of endoscope [12, 26]. According to my own experience and the report of the other authors [21], the duration of the endoscopic stapes surgery was similar to the procedures performed under the microscope.

Pure-tone audiograms demonstrated improved air- and bone conduction threshold averages across the three speech frequencies (0.5–1–2 kHz) 2 months after surgery (66.1 dB vs. 30.5 dB and 30.2 dB vs. 27.8 dB, respectively). The average postoperative ABG was within 10 dB in 12 ears and between 10 and 15 dB in the other eight ears compared to the 39.5 dB preoperative average ABG.

The CTN was preserved in all cases, and all but one patient described their postoperative taste function as being normal. One patient reported mild dysgeusia that resolved within 2 weeks. There were no patients with postoperative dysgeusia who underwent endoscopic stapedotomy by Kojima et al. [12], and temporary taste reduction in 1/15 (6.7 %) of the patients operated endoscopically was reported by Noguera et al. [21].

Rigid 3-mm diameter, 14-cm length endoscopes provide optimal illumination in addition to the possibility to work in such narrow field as external ear canal. However, a variety of sinonasal scopes that are already available in the departments can be used also successfully [12, 21, 26]. Special attention should be paid on prevention of excessive heating of the ear by the heat generated by the light source regardless of the sort of endoscopes [21]. Proper placing of the prosthesis can be difficult, especially in the first cases, and if done improperly, it may result in postoperative vertigo [21]. The use of microscope can prevent this situation.

Many authors recommend preservation of CTN whenever possible, especially if surgery is bilateral [4, 9–11, 14, 28]. Bilateral CTN damage can result in transient or permanent bilateral ageusia of the anterior two-thirds of the tongue, as well as a decreased resting salivary flow rate. Moreover, the patients may suffer from transient or persistent, distressing xerostomia or tactile dysgeusia [3, 11, 16]. Several authors stressed that the cutting of the CTN results in greater and more long-lasting taste dysfunction than the manipulation of the nerve [14, 28]. There are many unreported known as well as unrecognized divisions or injuries to the CTN. Indeed, some surgeons consider alteration in taste to be a minor postoperative problem, thus making it one that is probably underestimated.

TES is a safe and elegant procedure that is technically possible only for highly skilled otosurgeons. Comprehensive knowledge of standard stapedotomy techniques is obligatory before embarking on an endoscopic stapedotomy. In some occasions, the surgeon had to use microscope in the endoscopic surgery unexpectedly. Cerebrospinal fluid (CSF) gusher is a very rare (1/1000) and challenging event in ear surgery since its consequences for hearing can be dramatic [5]. Several authors described how to deal with this alarming situation that can end up with postoperative total hearing loss, vertigo, pneumocephalus, secondary meningeal infections, and even transient neurologic deficit [2, 5, 6, 22, 24]. The estimated incidence of floating footplate during stapes surgery is 2–5.8 % [1, 7, 27]. CSF gusher and floating footplate are usually unpredictable, and both involve serious consequences concerning not only the continuation of the surgical procedure but also the postoperative outcome. The surgeon has to know all the options of the treatment when confronted with these situations requiring bimanual quick management to prevent hearing deterioration and vertigo. Immediate switch to the microscope can be essential; thus, microscope should be routinely available in the operating room.

The TES can be beneficial in improving the visibility and accessibility of the stapes and the OWN, avoiding manipulation of the CTN and blind fracture of the stapedial crura. However, the main limitation of a TES is that it is a difficult one-hand surgery. Otosurgeons routinely look directly and binocularly into the operated ear through the otomicroscope and use both hands for the eradication of the pathology, suctioning, hemostasis, and subsequent reconstruction surgery; one hand is occupied with the endoscope and another performs other manipulations during ES [21]. In addition, the endoscopic surgeon watches a monitor, and this can result in a loss of depth perception that is later compensated with greater experience [21]. Assistance in using the operating microscope can be required when there is the need for two-hand manipulations for proper placing and coupling of the prosthesis, especially during the surgeon's initial endoscopic procedures.

TES requires previous training in performing simpler endoscopic procedures, such as myringoplasty or ossicular chain reconstruction. In inexperienced hands, the endoscopic approach can be associated with complications due to direct trauma from the tip of the endoscope to the facial nerve and to the ossicular chain. Finally, to a right-handed surgeon, the axis of work can be initially more comfortable when performing surgery on right ears. The relative difficulty in creating a hole in the footplate and positioning the prosthesis in left ears could be overcome with more training. The surgeon can feel some discomfort when changing endoscope to microscope despite stereoscopic vision provided by the microscope since the view of the ME structures becomes remarkably worse. However, this changing to the microscope can be necessary for safe proceeding/completion of surgery.

In summary, the use of endoscopes gives the surgeon better visualization of structures that are parallel to the axis of the microscope. Transcanal fully endoscopic stapedotomy is a feasible and safe technique for surgical management of hearing loss associated with otosclerosis. The favorable surgical and audiometric outcome of this technique indicates the worthiness of endoscopic approach in surgical armamentarium. The TES can be utilized in patients with unfavorable external or middle ear anatomy, in candidates for revision or bilateral stapedotomy, in patients with already impaired taste sensation, with food-, smell-, or taste-related occupations, and in those for whom the taste of food contributes appreciably to their quality of life. In cases of excessive bleeding, CSF gusher, floating footplate, difficulties with prosthesis placing, and other obstacles, it could be better to switch to microscope, which should be a part of the routine setting in middle ear surgery.

Financial Disclosure None

Conflict of Interest None

References

1. Ayache D, Sleiman J, Tchuente AN, Elbaz P. Variations and incidents encountered during stapes surgery for otosclerosis. Ann Otolaryngol Chir Cervicofac. 1999;116:8–14 [Article in French].
2. Cassano P, Decandia N, Cassano M, Fiorella ML, Ettorre G. Perilymphatic gusher in stapedectomy: demonstration of a fistula of internal auditory canal. Acta Otorhinolaryngol Ital. 2003;23:116–9.
3. Chen JM, Bodmer D, Khetani JD, Lin VV. Tactile dysgeusia: a new clinical observation of middle ear and skull base surgery. Laryngoscope. 2008;118:99–103.
4. Clark MP, O'Malley S. Chorda tympani nerve function after middle ear surgery. Otol Neurotol. 2007;28: 335–40.
5. Couvreur P, Baltazart B, Lacher G, Filippini JF, Vincey P. Perilymphatic effusion as a complication of otosclerosis. Rev Laryngol Otol Rhinol (Bord). 2003;124:31–7 [Article in French].
6. Flood LM, Kemink JL, Kartush JM. Pneumocephalus following treatment of a stapes gusher. Am J Otol. 1985;6:508–11.
7. Gierek T, Klimczak-Gołab L, Zbrowska-Bielska D, Majzel K, Witkowska M. Results of stapedotomy in the cases of "floating footplate". Otolaryngol Pol. 2005;59:263–6 [Article in Polish].
8. Gołabek W, Szymański M, Siwiec H, Morshed K. Incus subluxation and luxation during stapedectomy. Ann Univ Mariae Curie Sklodowska Med. 2003;58:302–5.
9. Guder E, Böttcher A, Pau HW, Just T. Taste function after stapes surgery. Auris Nasus Larynx. 2012;39: 562–6.
10. Guinand N, Just T, Stow NW, Van HC, Landis BN. Cutting the chorda tympani: not just a matter of taste. J Laryngol Otol. 2010;124:999–1002.
11. Just T, Homoth J, Graumüller S, Pau HW. Taste disorders and recovery of the taste function after middle ear surgery. Laryngorhinootologie. 2003;82:494–500 [Article in German].
12. Kojima H, Komori M, Chikazawa S, Yaguchi Y, Yamamoto K, Chujo K, et al. Comparison between endoscopic and microscopic stapes surgery. Laryngoscope. 2014;124:266–71.

13. Lesinski SG. Causes of conductive hearing loss after stapedectomy or stapedotomy: a prospective study of 279 consecutive surgical revisions. Otol Neurotol. 2002;23:281–8.
14. Mahendran S, Hogg R, Robinson JM. To divide or manipulate the chorda tympani in stapedotomy. Eur Arch Otorhinolaryngol. 2005;262:482–7.
15. Malafronte G, Filosa B. Fisch's reversal steps stapedotomy: when to use it? Otol Neurotol. 2009;30:1128–30.
16. Mandel L. Hyposalivation after undergoing stapedectomy. J Am Dent Assoc. 2012;143:39–42.
17. Michael P, Raut V. Chorda tympani injury: operative findings and postoperative symptoms. Otolaryngol Head Neck Surg. 2007;136:978–81.
18. Migirov L, Shapira Y, Horowitz Z, Wolf M. Exclusive endoscopic ear surgery for acquired cholesteatoma: preliminary results. Otol Neurotol. 2011;32:433–6.
19. Migirov L, Wolf M. Endoscopic transcanal stapedotomy: how I do it. Eur Arch Otorhinolaryngol. 2013;270:1547–9.
20. Miuchi S, Sakagami M, Tsuzuki K, Noguchi K, Mishiro Y, Katsura H. Taste disturbance after stapes surgery – clinical and experimental study. Acta Otolaryngol Suppl. 2009;562:71–8.
21. Nogueira Júnior JF, Martins MJ, Aguiar CV, Pinheiro AI. Fully endoscopic stapes surgery (stapedotomy): technique and preliminary results. Braz J Otorhinolaryngol. 2011;77:721–7 [Article in English, Portuguese].
22. Papadaki E, Prassopoulos P, Bizakis J, Karampekios S, Papadakis H, Gourtsoyiannis N. X-linked deafness with stapes gusher in females. Eur J Radiol. 1998; 29:71–5.
23. Poe DS. Laser-assisted endoscopic stapedectomy: a prospective study. Laryngoscope. 2000;110(5 Pt 2 Suppl 95):1–37.
24. Rebol J. The unilateral stapes gusher. Wien Klin Wochenschr. 2004;116 Suppl 2:90–2.
25. Saito T, Manabe Y, Shibamori Y, Yamagishi T, Igawa H, Tokuriki M, et al. Long-term follow-up results of electrogustometry and subjective taste disorder after middle ear surgery. Laryngoscope. 2001;111(11 Pt 1):2064–70.
26. Sarkar S, Banerjee S, Chakravarty S, Singh R, Sikder B, Bera SP. Endoscopic stapes surgery: our experience in thirty two patients. Clin Otolaryngol. 2013;38:157–60.
27. Szymański M, Gołabek W, Morshed K, Siwiec H. The influence of the sequence of surgical steps on complications rate in stapedotomy. Otol Neurotol. 2007;28:152–6.
28. Yung M, Smith P, Hausler R, Martin C, Offeciers E, Pytel J, et al. International common otology database: taste disturbance after stapes surgery. Otol Neurotol. 2008;29:661–5.

9 Middle Ear Implantation in Stapes Fixation

Maurizio Barbara, Luigi Volpini, and Simonetta Monini

9.1 Introduction: Clinical and Audiological Principles

The active middle ear implants (AMEI) are nowadays available for restoring the hearing impairment caused by middle ear pathology. Previous reports have been stressing the benefit that the AMEI may provide when, in case of external or middle ear diseases due to malformations or sequels from chronic otitis media, the use of conventional hearing aids (HA) is impeded [1–3]. The AMEI can be coupled to an intact ossicular chain, to a single ossicle, or to the middle/inner ear interfaces [footplate, round window (RW) membrane] and are able to deliver, via the actuator, the mechanical energy as a vibration for the cochlear stimulation, with 1–5 μm deflection amplitudes equivalent, at the low and medium frequencies, to roughly 120–130 dB SPL [4]. This electromechanical modality of cochlear stimulation is actually characterizing all the AMEI and represents the prerogative for their preferable use in case of a limited or disturbing effect of the HA, such as it may occur when the sound stimulation needs to be amplified in excess. Moreover, the AMEI would be of particular benefit when the bone conduction (BC) threshold is impaired, since they would be able to restore at the same time both the conductive (as air-bone gap) and the sensorineural component (BC threshold) contrary to an implantable BC device (BCI) that, in these circumstances, may reveal inadequate.

Stapes fixation represents a pathological finding in common with a few middle/inner ear disorders of more or less frequent observation (otosclerosis, tympanosclerosis, malformations, osteogenesis imperfecta, Paget's disease, and Thies Reis syndrome). From an audiological point of view, in these clinical entities the hearing function over time shows to differ. In addition, in the case of a systemic etiology (osteogenesis imperfecta, Paget's disease, and Thies Reis syndrome), any surgical option should be cautiously considered.

Otosclerosis represents an osteodystrophic, progressive process of the otic capsule in which the hearing function usually changes as natural course of the disease. In fact, after a first stage with a purely conductive hearing loss and a progressively increasing width of the air-bone gap, the BC threshold tends, in most of the cases, to progressively decline due to a more or less aggressive involvement of the inner ear at the level of the cochlea. This consideration is therefore conditioning the therapeutical approach where stapes surgery still plays a major role, being able to restore the hearing function close to normality in most of the cases that show a normal

M. Barbara (✉) • L. Volpini • S. Monini
NESMOS Department, ENT Clinic,
Sapienza Rome, Rome, Italy
e-mail: maurizio.barbara@uniroma1.it; luigi.volpini@gmail.com; simonetta.monini@uniroma1.it

I. Sziklai (ed.), *Surgery of Stapes Fixations*, DOI 10.1007/978-3-319-28576-4_9

or near-normal cochlear function, i.e., BC thresholds within 5–10 dB HL at all frequencies. Contrarily, when the BC threshold is below the normal range, and especially at the high-frequency level, the postoperative hearing function, even in the best operated cases, may result insufficient to cope with listening in particular situations (e.g., noisy environments), especially in the frequent case of a bilateral involvement.

Tympanosclerosis represents a hyaline degeneration of the eardrum/middle ear connective tissue, with calcific deposits that may localize in different sites, but produce evident auditory symptoms when the functional areas get involved. In this regard, the localization at the level of the oval window, with stapes fixation, and of the round window (RW), with its obliteration, may induce a hearing loss of different degree which is mostly conductive in the beginning.

A similar audiological pattern can also be found in case of *congenital* stapes fixation that, present since birth, may display a bilateral involvement and other associated anomalies (e.g., abnormal facial nerve course), although the hearing loss tends to remain stable, at least for a long time.

Osteogenesis imperfecta is a rare, genetically based heterogeneous group of diseases of the connective tissue that, once affecting the ear, may cause hearing loss that, when combined with bone fragility and blue sclerae, forms the classic triad known as Van der Hoeve syndrome [5]. Most frequently, a conductive or mixed type of hearing loss is found. While the fixation of the stapes footplate could usually be responsible for the conductive component, the pathogenesis of the sensorineural component of the mixed hearing loss is thought to be related to an anomalous bone formation inside and around the cochlea.

In the clinical practice, when the hearing loss caused by stapes fixation goes beyond the fence of a purely conductive form, the ear surgeon uses to implement the patient's counseling informing him/her on the possible need of wearing an external amplifying device even after a successful surgery. A similar situation will be displayed by those patients who, never operated before, develop a particularly rapid form of the disease, with the BC threshold more or less rapidly declining down to nearly not-measurable levels while eventually maintaining an air-bone gap. Also in these cases, the conventional stapes surgery can still be an option, but it will never provide a successful hearing outcome unless an external HA is successively adopted. Coming to this end, it is important to consider:

- A possible limitation of the conventional HA to amplify sounds in severe hearing loss, without causing distortion effects (feedback, occlusion, etc.)
- Local impediments to wear the HA, due to an external ear canal stenosis or chronic inflammation
- And, ultimately, the cosmetic and stigmatic aspect that, solved by stapes surgery, should again be taken into account by the patients

Under these circumstances, an AMEI could play a significant role, since most of them leave both the ear canal and the auricle free, can have a retroauricularly concealed external component (if not completely invisible), and differ from the conventional HA because they deliver a mechanical rather than an acoustic input to the cochlea, hence with less likelihood of distortion phenomena.

In terms of clinical presentations, different scenarios related to the different origin of stapes fixation can be observed. As aforementioned, the congenital form of stapes fixation tends to be stable over time as a purely conductive hearing loss, while the shifting to a mixed type of hearing loss is more likely to occur in the otosclerotic and tympanosclerotic (and genetic) forms. In these circumstances, it is possible to distinguish different audiometric patterns in:

1. Nonoperated ears:
    - BC thresholds within 35–40 dB that may be rehabilitated with conventional surgery or a BCI

  - BC thresholds below 45 dB, for which a BCI could reveal of limited efficacy
  - BC thresholds just measurable at the lowest audiogram levels, such as in the far-advanced otosclerosis [6], for which a cochlear implant could be indicated
  - Nonmeasurable BC thresholds, and a positive family history, such as in the very far-advanced otosclerosis [7], similarly treatable with cochlear implantation
2. Operated ears, with an initial, persistent favorable outcome, followed by a hearing decline that leads to a purely sensorineural or to a mixed, prevalently sensorineural, audiometric pattern

Before taking into consideration the experimental and clinical contributions that have appeared in the recent literature on the use of the AMEI for stapes fixation, a brief description of the AMEI that are, at the present time, available and appropriate for this purpose will be presented.

9.2 AMEI

The possible solutions include:

- Semi-implantable systems:
  - Vibrant Soundbridge or VSB® (Medel, Innsbruck, Austria)
  - Middle Ear Transducer or MET® (Cochlear, Melbourne, Australia)
  - Direct Acoustic Cochlear System or Codacs® (Cochlear, Melbourne, Australia)
- Fully implantable systems:
  - Carina® (Cochlear, Melbourne, Australia)

Intuitively, semi- and fully implantable devices do differ, the latter being completely implanted subcutaneously and therefore invisible, while the semi-implantable systems encompass an external component that is magnetically coupled, via the intact skin, to the internally positioned component.

9.2.1 Vibrant Soundbridge

The VSB® uses the electromagnetic modality of mechanical stimulation in order to deliver a vibratory effect on the ossicular chain (or a single ossicular element). It is composed of an external audio processor coupled via a magnet to the internal component, called VORP (Vibrating Ossicular Prosthesis) (Fig. 9.1). The audio processor contains two microphones, the electronics for the signal processing, the battery, and the magnet. The receiver unit in the VORP contains a demodulator circuitry that customizes the appropriate signal, in terms of power, to the patient' s hearing loss.

From the VORP extremity, a cable link departs to end up with a small magnetic drum-like component, called Floating Mass Transducer (FMT®), that represents the actuator to be put in contact in a single point with the selected middle ear structure (incus, stapes, footplate, round window membrane, promontory window). The FMT® is a solenoid (2.3 mm long, 1.6 mm width, weighing 25 mg) that includes two coils wrapped in a sealed housing, protected by a thin layer of resin for medical use. The last generation of VSB® for the RWM and the incus application presents some new features, such as a new signal processor, a shorter connector cable, new couplers, the

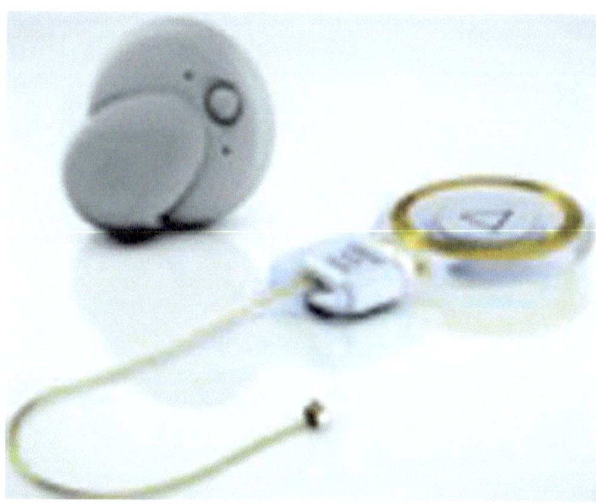

Fig. 9.1 The external (audio processor) and internal components (VORP and FMT) of the VSB

absence of the attachment clip, and, mostly, the MRI conditional at 1.5 T.

When planning a VSB® in the otosclerotic-operated subjects, the application can be performed on the long incus process, through a wide posterior tympanotomy in order to fully visualize the entire long incus process and the prosthesis assemblage down to the footplate. Another recent proposal involves, instead, both a coupler reinforcement of the standard incus vibroplasty or the VSB® placement on the short incus process, without performing the posterior tympanotomy, thus simplifying the surgical procedure that will be limited to the exposure of the posterior epitympanic space only [8, 9].

When a RWM coupling is planned, in accordance to the principles of an alternative cochlear stimulation that have been substantiated by Wever and Lawrence in the past [10], a wide posterior tympanotomy is required to give access to the middle ear cavity and to allow the thorough drill remodeling of the RW niche for the correct accommodation of the FMT®. It is possible to suggest that a RWM coupling could also be theoretically taken into consideration as primary procedure in case of stapedo-ovalar fixation, in alternative to the classic stapedotomy/stapedectomy.

9.2.2 MET®

This semi-implantable device, which is also based on the electromagnetic modality of mechanical stimulation, is composed of an external audio processor that contains the magnet, the battery, the digital sound processor, and the microphone, to be magnetically coupled to the implanted, internal component, which ends with an actuator, as a small probe rod-tip (Fig. 9.2).

When the ossicular chain after the primary stapes surgery looks mobile, the actuator can be placed in contact with the incus body, thus limiting the surgical procedure to the exposure of the entire epitympanic space. Also in this case, a possible alternative surgical placement would be the RWM. In this case, an enlarged mastoidectomy with a wide posterior tympanotomy is required, and specifically forged rod tips for the stapes, the oval window, and the RWM coupling will be used (Fig. 9.3).

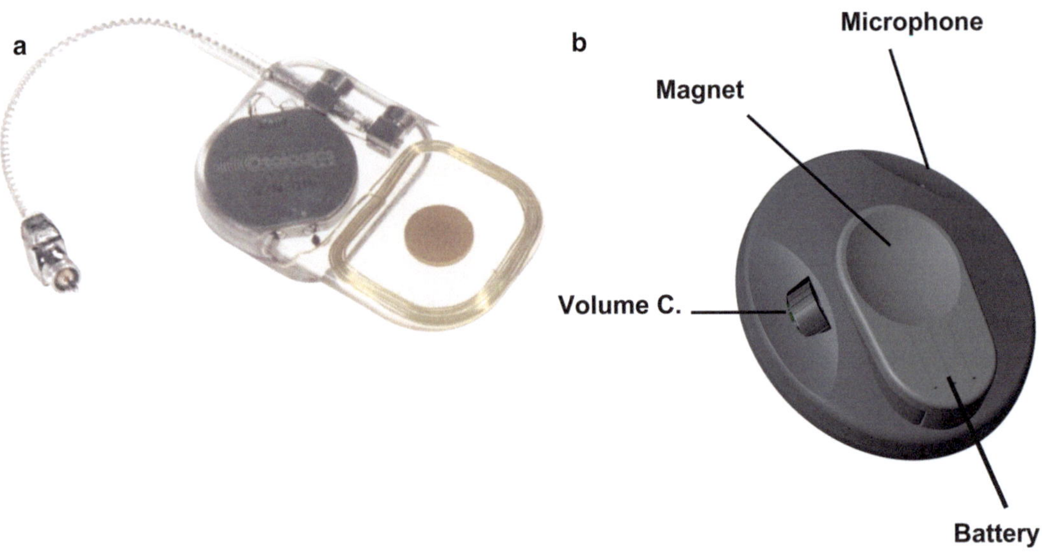

Fig. 9.2 The semi-implantable Middle Ear Transducer (MET). (**a**) Internal component (**b**) External component

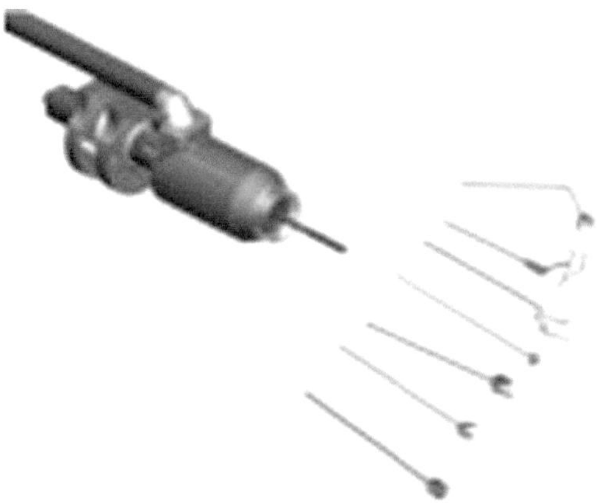

Fig. 9.3 MET/Carina transducer actuator, with the series of attachable tips for the different applications

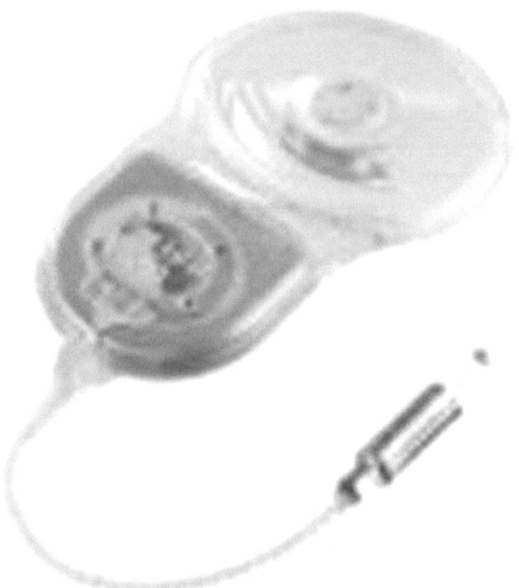

Fig. 9.4 The internal component of the Codacs

9.2.3 Codacs®

This semi-implantable device includes a BTE (behind the ear) unit that picks up the sound and contains the batteries, two microphones for directional hearing, and a digital signal-processing circuitry (Fig. 9.4). The Codacs® uses the electromagnetic modality of mechanical stimulation but delivers it as pressure waves directly to the cochlear fluids, via an artificial incus present at the actuator end, and that is connected to a titanium stapes prosthesis that protrudes into the vestibule. The surgical application includes a mastoidectomy with a wide posterior tympanotomy, where the neo-incus can be advanced up to the footplate region, in order to accommodate the piston prosthesis inside the hole performed through the footplate.

9.2.4 Carina®

This device represents, at the present time, the only fully implantable device that can be used for this purpose (Fig. 9.5). It is mostly similar to the semi-implantable version (MET®), differing due to its complete subcutaneous implantation. In the Carina® device, the microphone is implanted in a subcutaneous pouch and the internal battery needs to be recharged daily. The surgical procedure for the application on the incus body or the RWM coupling is similar to that described for the semi-implantable MET®.

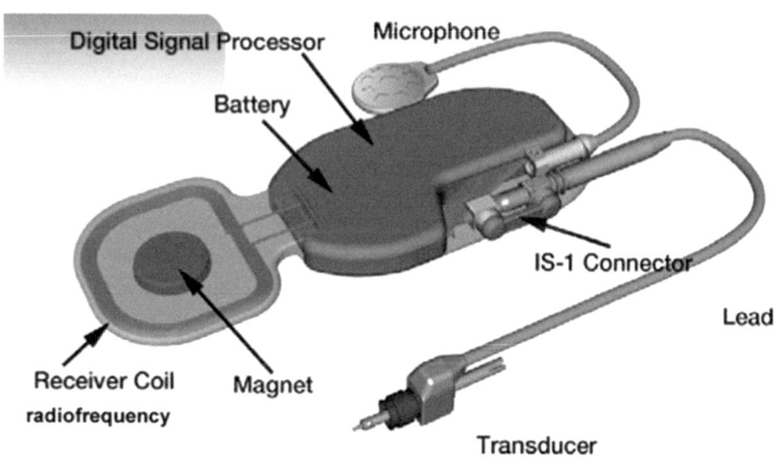

Fig. 9.5 The fully implantable Carina system

9.3 Experimental and Clinical Experiences

Due to the relatively recent introduction of the AMEI as an alternative to the conventional middle ear surgery or to a HA, the literature on the specific use of an AMEI for treating the stapes fixation is rather scanty. Otosclerosis is surely the more common cause for this problem and different clinical scenarios can be encountered:

- In the operated ears, it may be found:
  (a) *Stapes prosthesis correctly positioned, with a good ossicular chain motility*: the inner ear stimulation can be delivered either "empowering" this situation or stimulating the RWM.
  (b) *Stapes prosthesis correctly positioned, with a fixed ossicular chain*: the inner ear stimulation can be delivered by the ossicular chain, the RWM, or a promontory third window.
  (c) *Displaced stapes prosthesis*, with reclosure of the footplate hole: the stapes prosthesis can be repositioned correctly and then the surgery may proceed as in case (a).
- In the nonoperated ears:
  - In presence of stapes fixation, the inner ear stimulation can be obtained:
    (a) Combining the common stapedectomy with an AMEI
    (b) Via the round window membrane, with or without removal of the footplate and tissue sealing of the oval window
    (c) Directly on the fixed stapes/oval window region
    (d) Via a promontory bony window
    (e) With a direct inner ear fluid stimulation (Codacs®)

The RWM stimulation could therefore be considered an option in any case, operated or not, of stapes fixation. While coupling an AMEI to the RWM has been proved to be effective for rehabilitating a hearing impairment caused by chronic otitis media or its surgical sequels [11], the efficacy of the same mechanism with a fixed oval window is, at least theoretically, controversial. In this regard, Lupo et al. [12] have reproduced a laboratory model of stapes/oval window fixation and assessed electrophysiologically the RWM stimulation with a MET®. Similarly, Tringali et al. [13] have been performing the same study on animal models and found out that the RWM stimulation could also be effective in case of stapes fixation. Clinical data on a direct stimulation of the stapes/oval window region, in case of their fixation, are contrarily missing. Following a similar experimental protocol, Deveze et al. [14] have individuated and reproduced in fresh human cadaver temporal bones, different intraoperative situations that included:

- Stimulation of the stapes with footplate fixation
- Stimulation of the inner ear fluid through a stapedotomy, with and without fascia interposition

Interestingly, these investigators found that driving the oval window with a MET® on the interposed fascia could provide performances similar to the traditional incus coupling, and, even more surprisingly, a fair outcome could also be achieved when driving the stapes head in case of footplate fixation.

Another interesting, theoretically hazardous, application has been described in case of massive middle ear tympanosclerosis, which involves drilling of a bony niche for the FMT for its placement on the promontory wall [15]. This situation, which has also been experimentally tested on an animal model of stapes fixation, would eventually allow a discreet cochlear stimulation [16].

Considering that the AMEI should restore the hearing impairment in mixed hearing losses of severe degree, their output values should be of great importance. In this regard, an experimental study has taken into consideration the maximum output from several devices, showing that the Codacs® was providing a greater power in respect to a BCI or the VSB® [17].

In light of the abovementioned positive experimental results, some investigators have started to apply this option in the clinical practice.

9.3.1 Combined Stapes and AMEI Surgery (CSAS)

This procedure would theoretically allow, at the same time, to close the air-bone gap and to raise the BC threshold. It may be performed with some variants that regard:

- Timing: simultaneous or sequential (some months after the primary stapes surgery)
- Priority of placement: either AMEI first and piston prosthesis after (AFPA) or vice versa (PFAA)

This combined approach has been first described by Dumon [18], with a single case with the VSB® placed first (AFPA) (Fig. 9.6) and by Venail et al. [19] who presented four cases having differences in timing, approach, and device (both the VSB® and the MET®), warning on a possible labyrinthine reaction occurring after a simultaneous, PFAA procedure. In principle, the manipulation needed for the accurate coupling of the AMEI, when a piston prosthesis is already placed into the vestibule, is more likely to jeopardize the inner ear function. A similar experience, named as power stapes, has also been reported on a case of osteogenesis imperfecta with a severe, mixed hearing loss, by using a simultaneous AFPA procedure with the VSB® [20]. In line with this type of audiological indication, an additional device, the Codacs®, has been first experimentally [21] and thereafter clinically proven to be very efficient [22, 23].

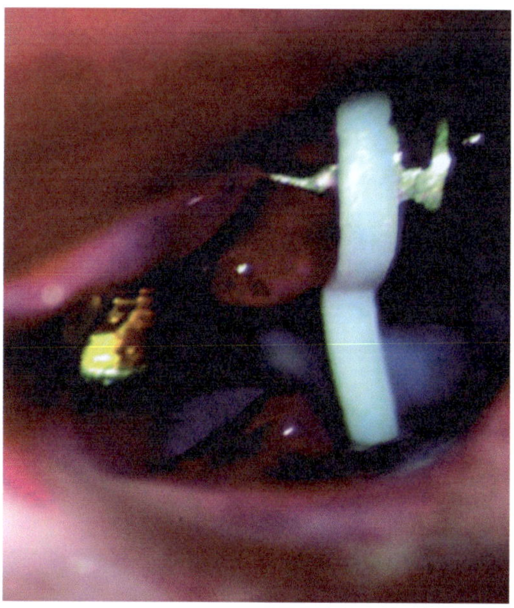

Fig. 9.6 A Teflon piston prosthesis is applied after the placement of the FMT on the long incus process (Courtesy of T. Dumon)

9.3.1.1 RW-Vibroplasty

Since the preliminary reports by Colletti et al. [11] of coupling the AMEI actuator on the RWM in conductive/mixed hearing loss due to chronic otitis media, further contributions ensued in regard to the RWM a coupling in case of stapes fixation mostly due to otosclerosis, using both the VSB® and the MET® devices [1, 3, 22, 24]. Beltrame et al. [3] have also commented on the lower amplification output of the RWM coupling in presence of a nonoperated, fixed stapes. As a matter of fact, this specific application could reveal of a certain interest if one wishes to decrease the risks of an inner ear damage, always possible when the stapes footplate is perforated. In this regard, animal and temporal bone experiments have shown that, even in this situation, an AMEI application could be advantageous [12, 13].

Conclusions

When, due to the stapes fixation of whatsoever etiology, a severe, mixed hearing loss is present, the optimal hearing rehabilitation cannot be achieved by applying the standardized surgical procedures only, but it may eventually be obtained by adding a further amplification. Considering the possible limitations of the conventional HA, in terms of inadequate amplification or incompatibility with local ear conditions (stenosis, chronic infections, etc.), it is possible to predict a future, beneficial role of the AMEI in these cases. The choice for the best surgical positioning, in this regard, will however only be derived by the validation of several clinical cases.

References

1. Dumon T, Gratacap B, Firmin F, Vincent R, Pialoux R, Casse B, Firmin B. Vibrant soundbridge middle ear implant in mixed hearing loss. Indications, techniques, results. Rev Laryngol Otol Rhinol (Bord). 2009;130:75–81.
2. Sargsyan S, Rahne T, Kösling S, Eichler G, Plontke SK. Hearing rehabilitation with single-stage bilateral vibroplasty in a child with Franceschetti syndrome. Eur Arch Otorhinolaryngol. 2014;271:1339–43.
3. Beltrame AM, Martini A, Prosser S, Giarbini N, Streitberger C. Coupling the vibrant soundbridge to cochlea round window: auditory results in patients with mixed hearing loss. Otol Neuro Otol. 2009;30:194–201.
4. Leysieffer H. Principle requirements for an electromechanical transducer for implantable hearing aids in inner ear hearing loss. I: technical and audiologic aspects. HNO. 1997;45:775–86.
5. Byers PH, Bonadio JF, Steinmann B. Osteogenesis imperfecta: update and perspective. Am J Med Genet. 1984;17:429–35.
6. House HP, Sheehy JL. Stapes surgery: selection of the patient. Ann Otol Rhinol Laryngol. 1962;70:1062–8.
7. Iurato S, Ettorre GC, Onofri M, Davidson C. Very far-advanced otosclerosis. Am J Otol. 1992;13:482–7.
8. Schraven SP, Dalhoff E, Wildenstein D, Hagen R, Gummer AW, Mlynski R. Alternative fixation of an active middle ear implant at the short incus process. Audiol Neuro Otol. 2014;19:1–11.
9. Mlynski R, Dalhoff E, Heyd A, Wildenstein D, Hagen R, Gummer AW, Schraven SP. Reinforced active middle ear implant fixation in incus vibroplasty. Ear Hear. 2015;36:72–81.
10. Wever E, Lawrence M. Physiological acoustics. Princeton: Princeton University Press; 1954.
11. Colletti V, Soli SD, Carner M, Colletti L. Treatment of mixed hearing losses via implantation of a vibratory transducer on the round window. Int J Audiol. 2006;45:600–8.
12. Lupo JE, Koka K, Holland NJ, Jenkins HA, Tollin DJ. Prospective electrophysiologic findings of round window stimulation in a model of experimentally induced stapes fixation. Otol Neuro Otol. 2009;30:1215–24.
13. Tringali S, Koka K, Holland NJ, Jenkins HA, Tollin DJ. Round window membrane implantation with an active middle ear implant: effects of performance of round window exposure and transducer tip diameter. Audiol Neuro Otol. 2010;15:291–302.
14. Deveze A, Koka K, Tringali S, Jenkins HA, Tollin DJ. Active middle ear implant application in case of stapes fixation: a temporal bone study. Otol Neuro Otol. 2010;31:1027–34.
15. Pau HW, Just T. Third window vibroplasty: an alternative in surgical treatment of tympanosclerotic obliteration of the oval and round window niche. Otol Neuro Otol. 2010;31:225–7.
16. Lupo JE, Koka K, Jenkins HA, Tollin DJ. Third-window vibroplasty with an active middle ear implant: assessment of physiologic responses in a model of stapes fixation in Chinchilla lanigera. Otol Neuro Otol. 2012;33:425–31.
17. Zwartenkot JW, Snik AFM, Mylanus EAM, Mulder JJS. Amplification options for patients with mixed hearing loss. Otol Neuro Otol. 2014;35:221–6.
18. Dumon T. Vibrant soundbridge middle ear implant in otosclerosis: technique – indication. Adv Otorhinolaryngol. 2007;65:320–2.
19. Venail F, Lavieille JP, Meller R, Deveze A, Tardivet L, Magnan J. New perspectives for middle ear implants: first results in otosclerosis with mixed hearing loss. Laryngoscope. 2007;117:552–5.
20. Kontorinis G, Lenarz T, Mojallal H, Hinze AL, Schwab B. Power stapes: an alternative method for treating hearing loss in osteogenesis imperfecta? Otol Neuro Otol. 2011;32:589–95.
21. Häusler R, Stieger C, Bernhard H, Kompis M. A novel implantable hearing system with direct acoustic cochlear stimulation. Audiol Neuro Otol. 2008;13:247–56.
22. Chatzimichalis M, Sim JH, Huber AM. Assessment of a direct acoustic cochlear stimulator. Audiol Neuro Otol. 2012;17:299–308.
23. Lenarz T, Verhaert N, Desloovere C, Desmet J, D'hondt C, González JC, Kludt E, Macías AR, Skarżyński H, Van de Heyning P, Vyncke C, Wasowski A. A comparative study on speech in noise understanding with a direct acoustic cochlear implant in subjects with severe to profound mixed hearing loss. Audiol Neuro Otol. 2014;19:164–74.
24. Martin C, Deveze A, Richard C, Lefebvre PP, Decat M, Ibañez LG, Truy E, Mom T, Lavieille JP, Magnan J, Dubreuil C, Tringali S. European results with totally implantable carina placed on the round window: 2-year follow-up. Otol Neuro Otol. 2009;30:1196–120.

10 Otosclerosis and Cochlear Implantation

Milan Profant, Zuzana Kabátová, and Lukáš Varga

Abbreviations

CBCT	Cone beam computed tomography
CI	Cochlear implantation
DACS	Direct acoustic cochlear stimulation
FAO	Far advanced otosclerosis
FN	Facial nerve
HRCT	High-resolution computed tomography
MRI	Magnetic resonance imaging
PTA	Pure tone audiometry
SNHL	Sensorineural hearing loss
UOHL	Unknown origin hearing loss

10.1 Otosclerosis and Cochlear Implantation

Cochlear implantation nowadays is a standard clinical tool to manage bilateral severe sensorineural hearing loss. Far advanced otosclerosis (FAO) is very frequently associated with severe hearing loss usually without any improvement with optimally fitted hearing aids. Thus cochlear implantation is fully indicated in FAO to improve hearing and communication skills.

The question is whether cochlear implantation is the only option in patients with some residual hearing in FAO. Van Loon et al. realised a meta-analysis of the published papers to evaluate the effect of stapedotomy in cochlear implant candidates with FAO [1]. They conclude that stapedotomy combined with hearing aid fitting results in a good outcome in a substantial amount of CI candidates with FAO. Stapedotomy should be attempted before considering CI in all patients with FAO. In patients with bilateral otosclerosis, a contralateral stapedotomy may offer patients the benefits of binaural processing. If bilateral stapedotomy yields an unsatisfactory outcome, the option for CI is still open. Calmels et al. present similar experience [2]. In a retrospective study, they evaluated 14 patients with nonmeasurable preoperative bone and air conduction thresholds and otosclerosis on temporal bone high-resolution CT scan. Stapes surgery followed by a well-fitted hearing aid was done in 11 patients and seven patients were implanted (including four patients who had poor results after stapedotomy). Objective and subjective results were statistically better in the cochlear implant group than in the stapedotomy group. However, four patients in the stapedotomy group had comparable results to the patients with cochlear implants.

Electronic supplementary material The online version of this chapter (doi:10.1007/978-3-319-28576-4_10) contains supplementary material, which is available to authorized users.

M. Profant (✉) • Z. Kabátová • L. Varga
Department of Otorhinolaryngology–Head and Neck Surgery, Faculty of Medicine and University Hospital, Comenius University, Antolska 11, Bratislava 85107, Slovakia
e-mail: profant@fnorl.sk

I. Sziklai (ed.), *Surgery of Stapes Fixations*, DOI 10.1007/978-3-319-28576-4_10

Lenarz et al. and Busch et al. presented first long-term results of a direct acoustic cochlear stimulator (DACS) [3, 4]. The DACS significantly improved hearing, speech intelligibility and satisfaction in patients with a severe-to-profound mixed hearing loss and can be considered a safe and useful alternative to conventional hearing aids. In the future the audiologic indications might be broadened also for the borderline candidates with FAO considered for CI.

Several papers confirmed optimal outcome of cochlear implantation in patients with deafness in FAO [5–9]. Nevertheless, there are several specific points in otosclerotic patients indicated for cochlear implantation to be discussed.

10.2 Pathophysiology of Otosclerosis

Remodelling of bone in the otic capsule of temporal bone is the characteristic feature of otosclerosis. These changes might be multifocal and may appear in any area of the otic capsule, most frequently in the oval and round window and along the cochlear duct. No other human bone shows otosclerotic changes. Otosclerotic changes may start as an inflammatory process with resorption of the bone. In this phase enchondral bone is resorbed by osteoclasts. Reasons for this early phase of otosclerotic changes are unknown. In the second phase, this bone is replaced by dysplastic immature basophilic bone, and the vascular areas are filled with connective tissue. In the next period, these structures are remodelled by losing part of the vasculature with maturation into the acidophilic bone. In the last phase, this area is getting sclerotised by mineralisation of the dysplastic bone growing into the dense compact bone [8]. If the stapes footplate area is involved in this process, annular ligament is getting calcified causing fixation of the stapes and developing conductive component of the hearing loss.

Involvement of the cochlear wall may be associated with the damage to the spiral ligament and vascular supply of the inner ear structures resulting in severe sensorineural impairment. Remodelling of otic capsule bone may also result in new bone formation in scala tympani or scala vestibuli with sensorineural deafness. In such a case, obstruction of the scala tympani might be a problem for inserting electrode array in a standard way.

10.3 Imaging of Otosclerosis for Cochlear Implantation

Imaging in FAO is an important part of the diagnostic process. Structural changes in the otic capsule may be seen on the HR (high-resolution) CT or CB (cone beam) CT. Demineralisation of the otic capsule bone shows the localisation of the otosclerotic foci, their size and relation to the scala tympani. Veillon et al. proposed classification of otosclerosis based on the size and localisation of the otosclerotic foci imaged by HRCT [10]:

Type IA: irregular thickened stapes footplate
Type IB: <1 mm focus anterior oval window region
Type II: >1 mm focus anterior oval window region
Type III: >1 mm focus anterior oval window region in contact with cochlear endosteum
Type IVA: extensive hypodense foci throughout middle layer of otic capsule (Fig. 10.1)
Type IVB: otic capsule involvement includes semicircular canals (Fig. 10.2)

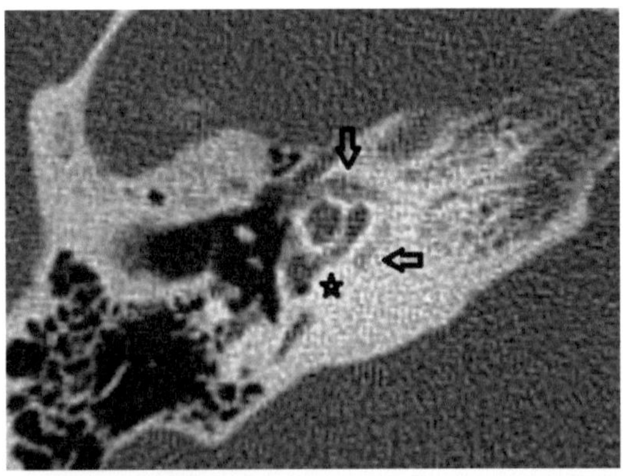

Fig. 10.1 Extensive hypodense foci throughout middle layer of otic capsule (*arrows*) (see narrowing of the basal turn of cochlea (asterisk))

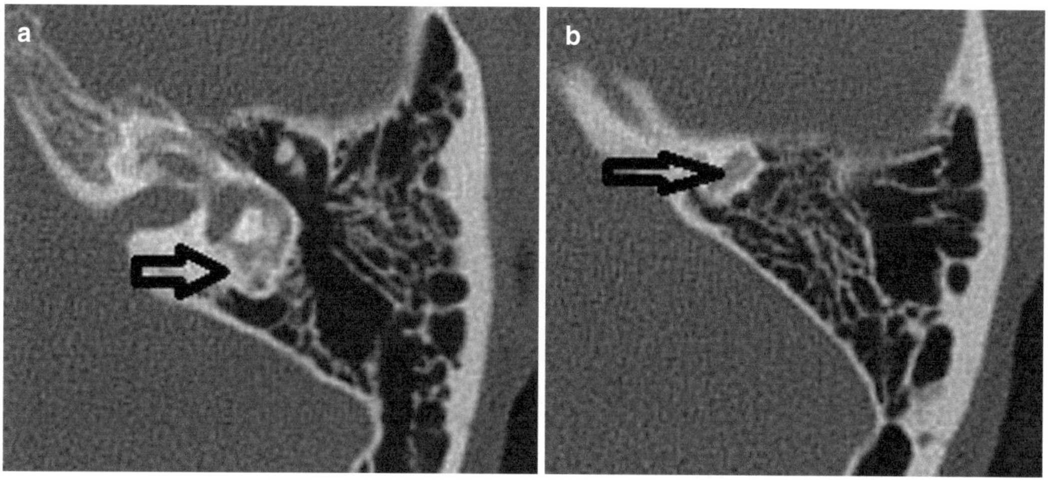

Fig. 10.2 (**a**, **b**) Involvement of otic capsule including semicircular canals. *Arrows* show otosclerotic foci in lateral (**a**) and anterior semicircular canal (**b**)

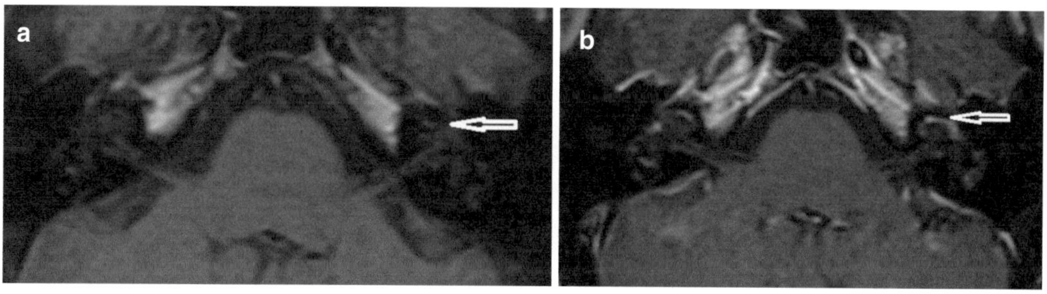

Fig. 10.3 (**a**, **b**) T1-weighted image (**a**) of cochlea with otosclerotic foci (*arrow*) and its enhancement after gadolinium contrast (**b**)

Extensive otosclerotic foci as it is shown in type IVB can be imaged also on MRI T1-weighted images with gadolinium contrast (Fig. 10.3).

Especially type IVA and type IVB may be associated with the severe sensorineural hearing loss and indication for the cochlear implantation. New bone formation and demineralisation throughout the otic capsule as it is presented in the types IVA and IVB may also be associated with a new bone formation inside the scala tympani, thus being an obstacle for electrode array insertion. Some authors demonstrated relation between the level of hearing loss and size and localisation of the otosclerotic foci on HRCT scan [11]. In our series of 72 patients, we have not confirmed this relationship. The advanced radiologic appearance of the otosclerotic foci did not correspond with the severity of hearing loss neither sensorineural nor conductive as it is shown in the bone conduction (Fig. 10.4) and air conduction threshold (Fig. 10.5) in PTA.

If cochlear implantation is indicated in FAO, MRI is highly recommended to image liquid in the cochlear canal in T2-weighted images which is the evidence of patency of this space.

10.4 Indications for CI in Far Advanced Otosclerosis and Selection of the Ear for CI

The hearing loss in severe otosclerosis can be subdivided into far advanced otosclerosis and very far advanced otosclerosis. Far advanced otosclerosis is defined by the audiogram with air

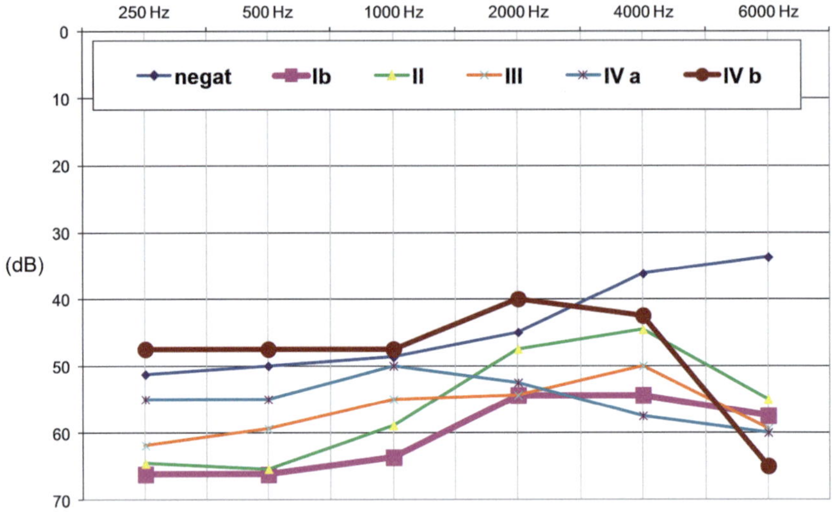

Fig. 10.4 Preoperative air conduction threshold (PTA) in the groups differentiated according to the radiological classification of otosclerosis (I–IVB)

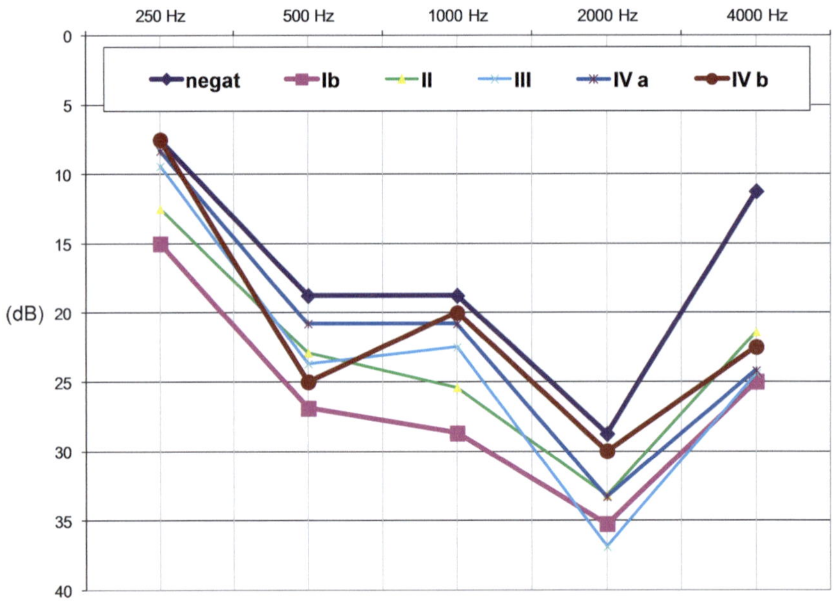

Fig. 10.5 Preoperative BC threshold (PTA) in the groups differentiated according to the radiological classification of otosclerosis (I–IVB)

conduction threshold 85 dB and more and nonrecordable bone conduction threshold. The term very far advanced otosclerosis is proposed to indicate otosclerotic patients with both bone and air conduction thresholds nonmeasurable on a standard clinical audiometer (blank audiogram) [12]. Despite the fact that audiologic criteria fulfilled the criteria for cochlear implantation, some of these patients may profit from stapedotomy and hearing aid. On the other hand, majority of these patients have already undergone stapes surgery, and deterioration of hearing might be the outcome of hearing loss progression or failure of the stapes surgery. In standard evaluation of unilateral cochlear implantation, usually the ear with shorter deafness duration is selected for the implantation. There are several papers to confirm negative correlation between deafness duration and postoperative performance [13]. Matterson et al. hold an opinion that it is the period of cortical deprivation rather than the duration of deafness in the auditory periphery which is the main determinant of speech perception [14]. In their paper, they confirmed that duration of deafness makes a significant contribution to the speech perception score 3 months after CI but then it ceases to exert an effect. Therefore the preference should not be given to implanting shortest deafened ear rather the preference should be given to implantation of the worse hearing ear.

10.5 Surgery in Cochlear Implantation

In majority of the cases, surgical procedure for cochlear implantation in patients with deafness due to otosclerosis does not differ from the standard cases. Temporal bone in otosclerotic patients is usually extremely well pneumatised with well-differentiated anatomical structures. Surgical orientation is very precise. Fixed stapes is not a problem at all. Transmastoid approach is highly recommended (Video 10.1). Anatomical space in the area of the facial recess is well pneumatised and mastoid portion of the facial canal in some cases can be seen in between the air cells. Reliable opening of the facial recess brings the surgeon directly to the area of round window and promontory (Video 10.2). If the scala tympani is patent, filled with perilymph (preoperative MRI scan) standard or soft electrode can be easily inserted (Video 10.3). In case that CT shows massive otosclerotic changes throughout the petrosal bone, testing the insertion with probe electrode is recommended. In the situation of patent scala tympani and aggressive otosclerotic process throughout the whole otic capsule, perimodiolar electrode is highly recommended to reduce the risk of the facial nerve stimulation.

Once the scala tympani obliteration or partial obliteration or bony ingrowth is demonstrated by CT or MRI, the surgeon should have all kinds of electrodes at his/her disposal. Short electrode array is recommended in case the basal turn can be explored or drilled out. In case of full obliteration of the basal turn, split electrode can be used (Fig. 10.6). The surgical procedure is slightly modified. Incus is removed and the bony bridge to support short process of incus is removed to the level of the facial canal. This way the posterior part of the tympanic cavity is fully visible

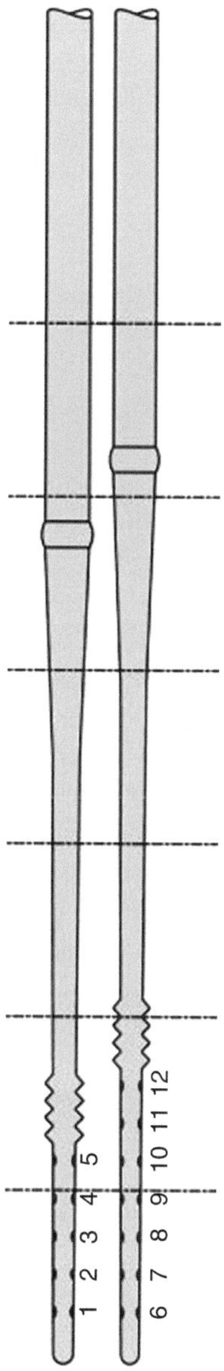

Fig. 10.6 Split electrode array for obliterated cochlea

through aditus and posterior tympanotomy. In the area of the basal turn of scala tympani, an opening for the first part of the split electrode is drilled out. The drilling is carried out in the direction of scala tympani (different orientation for the right and left side). Usually 6–8 mm of drilling is possible. Surgeon must be aware of the carotid canal position at the end of the drilling. In some cases drilling through the partially obliterated basal turn can open further part of the scala tympani which might be patent and ready for the short or standard electrode placement. If the drilled out canal is blind, the first part of the split electrode is accommodated in the preformed canal. The second turn of the cochlea projects to the area slightly below the cochleariform process. Drilling in this area is carried out in the similar way as standard cochleostomy. After opening the second turn of cochlear canal, the second part of the split electrode is inserted.

Intraoperative measurement of the acoustic nerve response from electrical stimulation is recommended. Stapedial reflex can also be seen as a contraction of the tendon despite the fact that the stapes is fixed. Since cochlear implantation in otosclerotic patients is always an implantation in postlingual adult patients, even if the intraoperative measurement is not done, the fitting procedure is relatively easy and reliable.

10.6 Results of CI in FAO

Several studies support the use of cochlear implants in FAO. Castillo et al. compared results of CI in patients with FAO and unknown origin hearing loss (UOHL) to the incidence of facial electrical stimulation and difficult insertion of the electrode array up to 3–5 years from surgery [15]. FAO patients achieved better results on the pure tone average and recognition of monosyllables. There were no differences towards complications. They conclude that CI in FAO has proven successful with results comparable to other similar cohorts and with low complications.

Semaan et al. compared hearing outcomes in patients with (FAO) undergoing cochlear implantation to an age-matched group of controls, to describe the effects of cochlear ossification on hearing [16]. Thirty patients with FAO were compared to 30 age-matched controls. In the FAO group, radiographic abnormalities were noted in 26.4 % of patients. There was no difference between the FAO and control groups in the mean short-term and long-term postoperative speech reception threshold, word and sentence scores. The presence of radiographic abnormalities did not predict hearing outcome. Intraoperative cochlear ossification was not associated with worse short-term word and sentence scores and for the long-term hearing outcome. In patients with FAO, effective and safe hearing rehabilitation can be accomplished with cochlear implantation.

Similar results in cochlear implantation in patients with FAO describe Muñoz-Fernández N et al. [17]. Out of 13 implantees with FAO, a total of three complications (problems) were found (implant failure, overstimulation of the facial nerve and bilateral tinnitus). One year after implantation, the average percentages of correct two-syllable words were 80 % and 85 % in open tests.

Rotteveel et al. analysed the speech perception performance of 53 cochlear implant recipients with otosclerosis to evaluate which factors influenced patients' performance [18]. The factors included disease-related data such as demographics, preoperative audiological characteristics, the results of CT scanning and device-related factors. The clinical presentation of the otosclerosis (rapid or slow progression) did not influence speech perception. Better performance was related to less severe signs of otosclerosis on CT scan, full insertion of the electrode array, little or no facial nerve stimulation and little or no need to switch off electrodes.

10.7 Complications and Problems of CI in Otosclerosis

Complication rate in patients after CI in FAO does not differ from those in standard CI in postlingually deaf patients. One of the postoperative problems might be the facial nerve stimulation

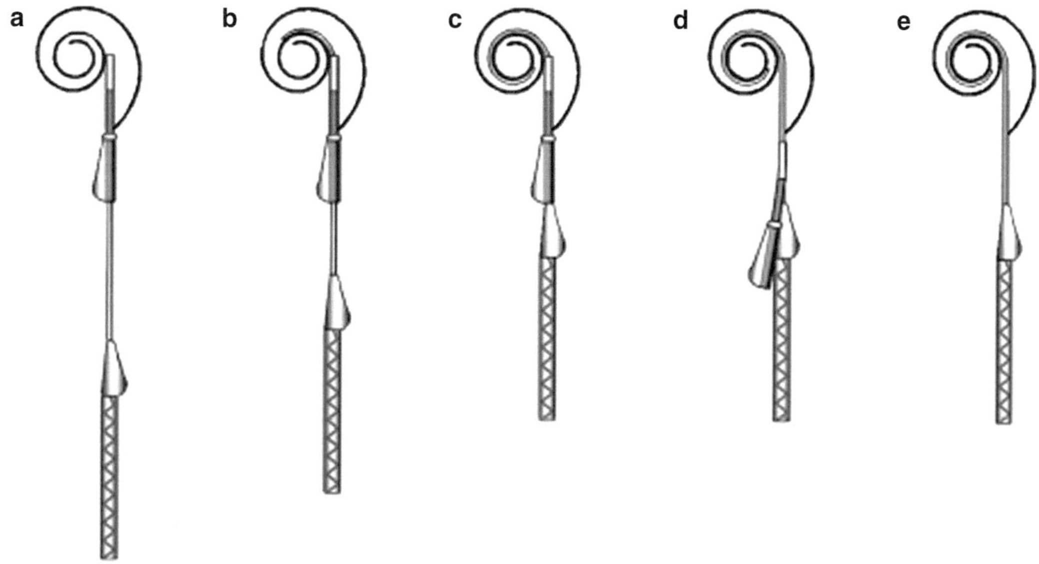

Fig. 10.7 Modiolus electrode for FAO to reduce risk of FN stimulation

by active cochlear implant. Facial nerve stimulation by cochlear implants occurs when advanced otosclerotic process invades the endosteum of both the upper basal turn of the cochlea and the facial nerve canal and all the bone between these two structures [19]. This may reduce impedance, shunting current to the facial nerve. The cause of FN stimulation has not been fully elucidated, and remarkable differences have been reported using different types of electrode arrays. After postmortem autopsy of 13 temporal bones with modiolar and straight electrodes, they conclude the FN stimulation occurs most commonly with straight electrode implants. This fact was also confirmed by Matterson et al. in the series of 59 patients with FAO. In the group of 35 patients implanted with the straight electrode, 14 experienced facial nerve stimulation [14]. On the other hand, in the group of 24 patients with perimodiolar electrode, no one experienced facial nerve stimulation.

Battmer et al. described four CI subjects with otosclerosis, who had been implanted with straight electrode between 9 and 12 years ago, suffering from severe FN stimulation [20]. The switch off of several contacts resulted in deteriorating speech understanding over time. Therefore, all subjects were reimplanted with a perimodiolar electrode. In all four cases, the postoperative fitting demonstrated no FN stim ulation on all electrodes up to maximum comfortable level. Electrodes with modiolar facing contacts and perimodiolar position reduce the possibility of facial nerve stimulation significantly due to more focused electrical stimulation (Fig. 10.7).

Conclusion

There is no doubt that cochlear implantation is a favourable option to manage severe sensorineural hearing loss in FAO. Results in speech perception and communication skills are comparable to those usually reached in other postlingual implantees. Optimal indication based on audiological criteria should be done taking into account some other options (preimplantation stapedotomy, contralateral stapedotomy and direct acoustic cochlear stimulation – DACS). Complication rate is very low usually associated with statistically acceptable device failure. Stimulation of the facial nerve may appear, and this phenomenon can be explained by the fact that extended otosclerotic process connects the endosteum of cochlear canal with the facial canal enabling the electrical current to stimulate facial nerve. New bone formation or scala tympani ossification may require special surgical technique and experienced surgeon. Imaging is extremely important to confirm patency of the scala tympani and size of the otosclerotic process. Both MRI and CT should be performed to get optimal information. Surgeon should have all kinds of electrodes available during the surgery. Intraoperative decision will select the appropriate type of electrode. In patients with advanced otosclerotic process throughout otic capsule confirmed by HRCT, perimodiolar electrode should be used to reduce the risk of facial nerve stimulation. Functional outcome of cochlear implantation in patients with far advanced otosclerosis, especially results in speech perception, and communication skills justify this indication.

References

1. van Loon MC, Merkus P, Smit CF, Smits C, Witte BI, Hensen EF. Stapedotomy in cochlear implant candidates with far advanced otosclerosis: a systematic review of the literature and meta-analysis. Otol Neurotol. 2014;35(10):1707–14.
2. Calmels MN, Viana C, Wanna G, Marx M, James C, Deguine O, Fraysse B. Very far-advanced otosclerosis: stapedotomy or cochlear implantation. Acta Otolaryngol. 2007;127(6):574–8.
3. Lenarz T, Zwartenkot JW, Stieger C, Schwab B, Mylanus EA, Caversaccio M, Kompis M, Snik AF, D'hondt C, Mojallal H. Multicenter study with a direct acoustic cochlear implant. Otol Neurotol. 2013;34(7):1215–25.
4. Busch S, Kruck S, Spickers D, Leuwer R, Hoth S, Praetorius M, Plinkert PK, Mojallal H, Schwab B, Maier H, Lenarz T. First clinical experiences with a direct acoustic cochlear stimulator in comparison to preoperative fitted conventional hearing aids. Otol Neurotol. 2013;34(9):1711–8.
5. Toung J, Zwolan T, Spooner T, Telian SA. Late failure of cochlear implantation resulting from advanced cochlear otosclerosis: surgical and programming challenges. Otol Neurotol. 2004;25(5):723–6.
6. Sainz M, Garcia-Valdecasas J, Ballesteros JM. Complications and pitfalls of cochlear implantation in otosclerosis: a 6-year follow-up cohort study. Otol Neurotol. 2009;30(8):1044–8.
7. Ramsden R, Rotteveel L, Proops D, et al. Cochlear implantation in otosclerotic deafness. Adv Otorhinolaryngol. 2007;65:328–34.
8. Ramsden R, Bance M, Giles E, Mawman D. Cochlear implantation in otosclerosis: a unique positioning and programming problem. J Laryngol Otol. 1997;111: 262–5.
9. Quaranta N, Bartoli R, Lopriore A, Fernandez-Vega S, Giagnotti F, Quaranta A. Cochlear implantation in otosclerosis. Otol Neurotol. 2005;26(5):983–7.
10. Veillon F, Stierle JL, Dussaix J, Ramos-Taboada L, Riehm S. Otosclerosis imaging: matching clinical and imaging data. J Radiol. 2006;87(11 Pt 2):1756–64.
11. Lagleyre S, Sorrentino T, Calmels MN, Shin Y, Escude B, Deguine O, Fraysse B. Reliability of high-resolution CT scan in diagnosis of otosclerosis. Otol Neurotol. 2009;30:1152–9.
12. Iurato S, Ettorre GC, Onofri M, Davidson C. Very far-advanced otosclerosis. Am J Otol. 1992;13(5):482–7.
13. Tyler RS, Summerfield AQ. Cochlear implantation: relationships with research on auditory deprivation and acclimatization. Ear Hear. 1996;17(3 Suppl): 38S–50.
14. Matterson AG, O'Leary S, Pinder D, Freidman L, Dowell R, Briggs R. Otosclerosis: selection of ear for cochlear implantation. Otol Neurotol. 2007;28(4):438–46.
15. Castillo F, Polo R, Gutiérrez A, Reyes P, Royuela A, Alonso A. Cochlear implantation outcomes in advanced otosclerosis. Am J Otolaryngol. 2014;35(5): 558–64.
16. Semaan MT, Gehani NC, Tummala N, Coughlan C, Fares SA, Hsu DP, Murray GS, Lippy WH, Megerian CA. Cochlear implantation outcomes in patients with far advanced otosclerosis. Am J Otolaryngol. 2012;33(5):608–14.
17. Muñoz-Fernández N, Morant-Ventura A, Achiques MT, Dualde-Beltrán D, Garcia-Callejo FJ, Monrroy-Parada MV, Pitarch I, Latorre E, Marco-Algarra J. Evolution of otosclerosis to cochlear implantation. Acta Otorrinolaringol Esp. 2012;63(4):265–71.
18. Rotteveel LJ, Snik AF, Cooper H, Mawman DJ, van Olphen AF, Mylanus EA. Speech perception after cochlear implantation in 53 patients with otosclerosis: multicentre results. Audiol Neuro Otol. 2010;15(2):128–36.
19. Seyyedi M, Herrmann BS, Eddington DK, Nadol Jr JB. The pathologic basis of facial nerve stimulation in otosclerosis and multi-channel cochlear implantation. Otol Neurotol. 2013;34(9):1603–9.
20. Battmer R, Pesch J, Stöver T, Lesinski-Schiedat A, Lenarz M, Lenarz T. Elimination of facial nerve stimulation by reimplantation in cochlear implant subjects. Otol Neurotol. 2006;27(7):918–22.

11 Revision Stapes Surgery

Roberto Filipo, M. Viccaro, and E. Covelli

11.1 Introduction

Despite, to date, stapedectomy and stapedotomy being considered as safe and reliable means of surgical correction of otosclerosis, surgical failures remain a recognized incidence [1–5].

The incidence of revision stapes surgery is about 10–20 % as reported in literature by Lambert and Meyer in 2004 [6].

The most frequent causes of revision stapes surgery are reported in Table 11.1 [7–13].

On the basis of the data reported in the literature, we note that in many cases, there is a greater variability of findings linked to the surgical technique performed. For example, a precise small fenestra with adequate depth of insertion (0.25/0.50 mm) probably prevents reclosing of the oval window and the risk of perilymphatic fistula. The fistula, in theory, can occur more easily in large fenestra or hemi-stapedectomy also with interposition.

Regarding middle ear fibrosis, we believe that it is necessary to evaluate during the follow-up of the patient the ventilation of the middle ear, intervening with medical or surgical nasal therapy when a slight tympanic retraction appears. Another possible cause of postoperative fibrosis is related to the erosion of the scutum or wrong repositioning of the flap or its tearing. Actually, the granulomatous reaction became very rare as an excessive chronic inflammation that forms tissue around the prosthesis and the oval windows. Although the etiology is uncertain, a different pathophysiological mechanism has been proposed and the main cause is a foreign body reaction to the material used in filling the oval windows.

The necrosis of the long process of the incus is often due to the type of prosthesis applied. In these cases the stabilization and reconstruction of the incus long process is possible by hydroxyapatite cement that would improve hearing results after the revision. In case of limited necrosis, a bended prosthesis can be applied.

11.2 Overview of Personal Cases

Coming to our experience (Table 11.2) that includes a period from 2000 to 2014, we can divide our cases in two groups:

1. Patients operated by us, unsatisfied in terms of auditory results, demanding a hearing improvement. In these cases we have the advantage of deeper knowledge of the previous surgical operation and the postoperative follow-up. Sometimes during the follow-up, it is possible to observe the evolution of the deafness with conductive or sensorineural hearing loss. In these cases we can propose a revision surgery or hearing aids or both.

R. Filipo (✉) • M. Viccaro • E. Covelli
Department of Otorhinolaryngology,
"Sapienza" University of Rome, Rome, Italy
e-mail: Roberto.filipo@uniroma1.it

I. Sziklai (ed.), *Surgery of Stapes Fixations*, DOI 10.1007/978-3-319-28576-4_11

Table 11.1 Most frequent causes of revision stapes surgeries in the literature

Author (years)	Displacement of the piston (%)	Incus necrosis (%)	Perilymphatic fistula (%)	Immobilization of the ossicular chain (%)	Obliteration of oval window (%)	Fibrous tissue (%)
Pedersen (1994)	22.5	11.2	3.2	–	16	–
Cokkeser et al. (1994)	32	34	–	–	16	23
Glassock et al. (1987)	40.3	21.2	7.5	–	12	–
Han et al. (1997)	58.1	43.	5.4	2.7	24.3	44.6
Lesinski (2003)	–	30	7	4	–	–
Fisch et al. (2001)	48.7 %	37.5	6.2	8.7 (tot) 37.5 (part)	15	30
De La Cruz and Fayad (2000)	52.8	25.8	–	0.8	14	–
Lippy et al. (2003)	–	34.6	–	7.5	2.7	–
Betsch et al. (2003)	–	8.5	–	–	7	–

Table 11.2 Causes of stapes revision surgery treated at our department in patients operated by us

Number of patients/causes	Displacement of the piston	Incus necrosis	Perilymphatic fistula	Immobilization of the ossicular chain	Obliteration of oval window	Fibrous adhesion
13	10 (77 %)	1 (8 %)	–	1 (8 %)	2 (15 %)	6 (46 %)

2. Patients operated in other hospitals that came to our observation due to probably unsatisfaction on the previous surgical treatment.

The clinical evaluation before the surgical revision is crucial. Audiology plays a strategic role in indication for revision surgery. The test battery utilized by our group is based on:

- Pure tone audiometry and tympanometry
- Speech audiometry with and without hearing aids
- Speech audiometry in noise

The accurate audiological evaluation allows us to consider the overall residual auditory function [14], the weight of the contralateral ear, and any sensorineural hearing loss arisen following the intervention that should be considered in the preoperative interview with the patient.

Radiology in the preoperative evaluation plays another important role. The high-resolution CT or preferably the cone beam combined with the other clinical data can provide specific information: the placement of the prosthesis with respect to the incus, incus necrosis, and conditions of the shaft with respect to the oval window. The cone beam can be very useful in those cases where the patient shows vertigo postoperatively; it can highlight as the prosthesis penetrates too deeply in the vestibule. The cone beam can also be used to visualize the content of the vestibule as air bubbles and bone fragments and radiological signs of perilymphatic fistula.

In the last 15 years, we have performed about 70 stapedotomy per year. Generally surgical revision procedures were performed under local anesthesia and conscious sedation in order to have the feedback of the patient during surgery. According to data presented in literature, our

Table 11.3 Causes of stapes revision surgery performed in our department in patients operated in other hospitals

Number of patients/ causes	Displacement of the piston	Incus necrosis	Perilymphatic fistula	Immobilization of the ossicular chain	Obliteration of the oval window	Fibrous adhesion	Prosthesis with no adequate connection with the incus
29	7	6	2	1	3	5	5

success rate in the revision surgery is little above 70 %. Out of more than 950 cases performed by us in this period, 13 are the cases that came to us for revision. This number could be probably higher if you consider that some of our stapedotomy cases went directly to other specialists for the follow-up.

The findings of our personal revisions are mainly based on displacement of the piston and middle ear fibrosis and adhesion.

As we already mentioned, the piston displacement is fundamentally due to a short piston or to cases of large fenestra with no adequate penetration of the shaft.

The second most frequent cause of revision surgery is the occurrence of adhesions or fibrosis that led us to consider carefully in the follow-up the nasal dysventilation of the middle ear.

The limited number of incus necrosis could be correlated to the type of prosthesis that has been used. We use platinum piston Audio® that allows the surgeon to perform adequate crimping without applying too much pressure on the bone.

I would like to add some comments regarding the surgical cases operated in other hospitals and revised by us (group 2, Table 11.3). The causes of failures are almost equally distributed. Few cases of perilymphatic fistula were observed, probably due to the fact that the patient came to us in stabilization of symptomatology (no vertigo and further deterioration of the auditory threshold).

In two cases of necrosis of the incus that has been revised by us, a bended prosthesis, Lippi type, has been used. In four cases of reconstruction of the incus long process, a hydroxyapatite cement has been used and worse results than the primary surgery were observed.

In the case of management of the middle ear fibrous adhesion, it is useful to use a Beaver thin knife or a fiber laser and the results observed were inconstant both short and long term, probably due to the loss of elasticity of the eardrum, and a tympanoplasty could be proposed.

Regarding the cases with prosthesis with no adequate connection with the incus (partially loose prosthesis), we made a better crimping or we substituted the prosthesis.

In conclusion, revision surgery requires a very complete patient counseling in terms of possible recovery. In elderly patients, especially in those with conductive (25/30 dB) and sensorineural hearing loss, an alternative therapy, based on hearing aid, could be considered. In our experience, these patients are frequently unsatisfied, even if correct surgery has been performed, due to the presence of the sensorineural hearing loss that influences the auditory perception, more than the conductive component. For these reasons a new operation does not change significantly the situation. Prior to the surgical revision, every case should be evaluated on the basis of the request of the patient and on the basis of what is possible to achieve with surgical intervention.

References

1. Massey BL, Kennedy RJ, Shelton C. Stapedectomy outcomes: titanium versus teflon wire prosthesis. Laryngoscope. 2005;115:249–52.
2. Krieger LW, Lippy WH, Schuring AG, Rizer FM. Revision stapedectomy for incus erosion: long-term hearing. Otolaryngol Head Neck Surg. 1998;119:370–3.
3. Sheehy JL, Nelson RA, House HP. Revision stapedectomy: a review of 258 cases. Laryngoscope. 1981;91:43–51.
4. De La Cruz A, Fayad JN. Revision stapedectomy. Otolaryngol Head Neck Surg. 2000;123:728–32.
5. Lippy WH, Battista RA, Berenholz L, Schuring AG, Burkey JM. Twenty-year review of revision stapedectomy. Otol Neurotol. 2003;24:560–6.

6. Meyer TA, Lambert PR. Primary and revision stapedectomy in elderly patients. Curr Opin Otolaryngol Head Neck Surg. 2004;12:387–92. Review.
7. Pedersen CB. Revision surgery in otosclerosis – operative findings in 186 patients. Clin Otolaryngol Allied Sci. 1994;19:446–50.
8. Cokkeser Y, Naguib M, Aristegui M, Saleh E, Landolfi M, Russo A, Sanna M. Revision stapes surgery: a critical evaluation. Otolaryngol Head Neck Surg. 1994;111:473–7.
9. Glasscock 3rd ME, McKennan KX, Levine SC. Revision stapedectomy surgery. Otolaryngol Head Neck Surg. 1987;96:141–8.
10. Han WW, Incesulu A, McKenna MJ, Rauch SD, Nadol Jr JB, Glynn RJ. Revision stapedectomy: intraoperative findings, results, and review of the literature. Laryngoscope. 1997;107:1185–92.
11. Lesinski SG. Revision stapedectomy. Curr Opin Otolaryngol Head Neck Surg. 2003;11:347–54.
12. Fisch U, Acar GO, Huber AM. Malleostapedotomy in revision surgery for otosclerosis. Otol Neurotol. 2001;22:776–85.
13. Betsch C, Ayache D, Decat M, Elbaz P, Gersdorff M. Revision stapedectomy for otosclerosis: report of 73 cases. J Otolaryngol. 2003;32:38–47.
14. De Seta E, Rispoli G, Balsamo G, Covelli E, De Seta D, Filipo R. Indication for surgery in otosclerotic patients with unilateral hearing loss. Otol Neurotol. 2009;30:1116–21.

12 Outcome Measures After Primary Surgery of Stapes Fixations

Istvan Sziklai

Independent of surgical technique, stapes prosthesis used, and postoperative care, some outcome measures guarantee the satisfaction of the patient. Anticipating the surgical intervention, a written consent from the patient is taken. This requires informing the patient about potential risks versus benefits of the surgery. Surgery of stapes fixations is performed in most cases without identification of the background disease. The etiology of the stapes fixation can only be verified by histological examination of the stapes footplate. It can be otosclerosis (in approximately 70 % of stapes fixation cases) but can be due to other abnormalities (inflammation, tympanosclerosis, calcification, amyloidosis, etc.), as well [1]. Actually, comprehensive studies are not available on postoperative hearing outcomes according to different abnormalities leading to stapes ankylosis. This means that a probability of hearing result after stapes surgery can only be predicted to the patient without sincere knowledge of an unexpected failure of the surgery. CT scanning can explore active otosclerosis which is a fragment of the (e.g., 50 %) stapes fixations causing conductive hearing loss. Anti-measles IgG serology in conductive hearing loss patients helps to identify otosclerosis [2]. As there is no evidence-based outcome measure of the surgical treatment of those stapes fixations which are caused by non-otosclerotic diseases, we should be prepared to counsel the patient about the possibility of unexpected minor or major failures of the surgery. Minor failures are unchanged hearing capacity, temporary dizziness, temporary facial weakness, temporary tinnitus, prolonged wound healing, and fullness sensation in the ear. Major complications are deafness, facial palsy, severe vertigo, perichondritis of the auricle, inflammation in the middle ear, and perforation of the tympanic membrane. We should keep in mind that approximately 1 % of stapedectomies result in total loss of inner ear function [3]. A written consent should clarify these details as to provide the patient with the possibility of decision to choose surgery for hearing improvement or other options, e.g., hearing aid. Differences in the risk of early and late postoperative complications between surgery of otosclerotic and non-otosclerotic stapes fixations are not yet published. In the era of laser-assisted stapedotomy, the risk of drop of a floating footplate into the vestibule is low. Stapedectomy significantly increases the possibility to cause floating footplate in non-otosclerotic stapes fixations. The adhesion between the oval window and the stapes footplate is tight in otosclerosis (Fig. 12.1). Non-otosclerotic fixations produce bulky footplate edges toward the annular ligament, but the interface between the footplate and the oval window

I. Sziklai
Department of Otorhinolaryngology and Head and Neck Surgery, Debrecen University, Debrecen, Hungary
e-mail: isziklai@med.unideb.hu

I. Sziklai (ed.), *Surgery of Stapes Fixations*, DOI 10.1007/978-3-319-28576-4_12

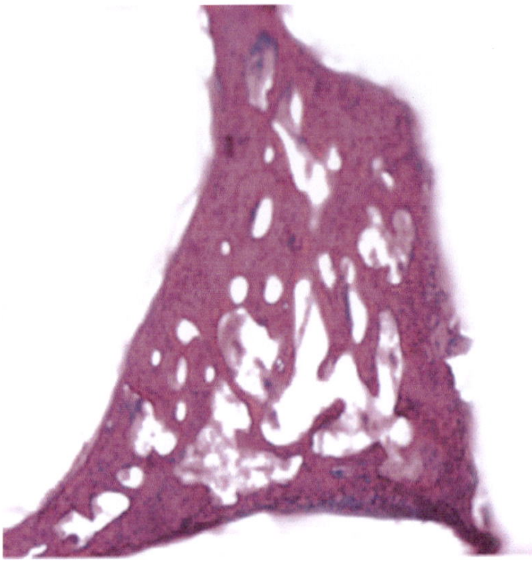

Fig. 12.1 Otosclerotic stapes footplate. Right is the anterior pole of the footplate. Upper aspect is the anterior crus. Note the broken surface toward the annular ligament as a sign of a tight adhesion of the footplate to the oval window. Hematoxylin-eosin staining. Magnification is 70× (From the collection of T. Karosi)

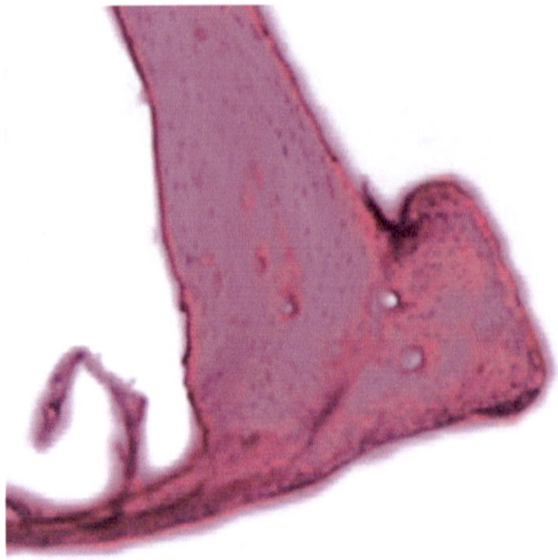

Fig. 12.2 Non-otosclerotic deformity of the stapes footplate due to extensive calcification. The anterior pole (*right*) facing toward the annular ligament has a smooth surface but bulky. Hematoxylin-eosin staining. Magnification is 70× (From the collection of T. Karosi)

is smooth (Fig. 12.2). Fragmentation of the footplate in non-otosclerotic fixations may lead to mobilization of the footplate pieces and their being sunk in the vestibular perilymph. This is rare because the perilymph outflow and the surface tension of the fluid work against it. When it happens, however, sensorineural hearing loss or deafness can develop. The small-hole technique decreases the risk of floating footplate to a negligible level. CO_2 laser for fenestration of the footplate has been proven superior over the conventional manual techniques by decreasing the incidence of stapes footplate fracture or sensorineural hearing loss [4].

Irrespective of the surgical technique, stapedectomy or stapedotomy, some prognostic factors can be collected for the prediction of the surgical outcome and functional results [5]:

1. Anomaly in the course of the facial nerve (dehiscent canal, prominent position)
2. Shape of the external auditory meatus (narrow, curved)
3. Aberrant incus long process
4. Visibility of the stapes footplate (deep)

Some additional, surgery-related technical items determine the prognostics of the surgery and the hearing result:

1. Suction around the oval window after opening the vestibule causes sensorineural hearing loss or deafness.
2. Bloodless oval window makes possible the correct orientation of the piston.
3. Fixation of the piston to the long process of the incus should be tight enough.
4. Integrity of the tympanic membrane is necessary to prevent middle ear infection.

Combination of 2–3 of these abnormalities in the surgical field or irrespecting the technical rules can lead to unexpected complication/s or poor functional outcome, postoperatively.

12.1 Hearing Outcome After Stapedectomy/Stapedotomy

The surgically obtained hearing improvement is calculated by comparison of preoperative air and bone conduction pure tone thresholds and air-bone gap to the early (<1 month) and late

Table 12.1 Postoperative hearing improvement after stapedectomy (PTA: 0.5-1-2/3 kHz) as to air conduction gain, bone conduction change, or air-bone gap

	Early (<1 month)	Late (1 year)	Late (3–10 years)
Air conduction gain dB	15 [6]	33.5 [7], 27 [6]	31.3 [7]
Bone conduction change, dB		10 [7]	9.1 [7]
Air-bone gap, dB	23 [6], 0–10 (44 % of cases) [8]	6 [6], 0–10 (54 % of cases) [8]	0–10 (58 % of cases) [8]

Table 12.2 Postoperative hearing results after stapedotomy (PTA: 0.5-1-2-3 kHz)

	Early	Late (1 year)	Late (3–10 years)
Air conduction gain, dB		26.5 [7], 24.2 [9]	25.7 [7], 26.1 [9]
Bone conduction change or preop/postop, dB		4.7 [7], 25.8/24 [9]	4.6 [7], 25.8/25.2 [9]
Air-bone gap (preop/postop), dB	0–10 (38 % of cases) [8]	25.6/1.7 [9], 0–10 (58 % of cases) [8]	0–10 (52 % of cases) [8]

Table 12.3 Influence of stapedectomy and stapedotomy on bone conduction change in 4 kHz (positive numbers are threshold elevations; negative numbers are threshold improvements) and on air conduction in 8 kHz

	Early: 4 kHz, dB	Late (1 year): 4 kHz, dB	Late (3–10 years), 4 kHz, dB	Early: 8 kHz (air) dB	Late. 8 kHz (air) dB	Late (10 years), 8 kHz, dB
Stapedectomy: piston	6 [10], 6 [11], 6.31 [14]	0.4 [7], 3 [10], 0.3 [5], 3.2 [14]	−3.5 [7]	8 [10], 8 [14]	4 [10], 7.1 [15], 4.2 [14],	7.9 [12]
Stapedotomy: 0.4 mm hole		0.6 [9]	3.8 [9]			
Stapedotomy: 0.6 mm hole	7.1 [13]	2.5 [7]	1.3 [7]			

(>1 year) postoperative air and bone conduction thresholds and air-bone gap (Tables 12.1 and 12.2). The very early postoperative threshold shift (within 7 days) in speech frequencies improves after 1 month.

The early thresholds and the air-bone gap reflect the eligibility of the surgical technique. Improvement in the bone conduction threshold envisions the Carhart effect. Late postoperative threshold shift after 1 year is stabilized and a gold standard for stapes surgery is a postoperative hearing result less than 30 dB air conduction pure tone threshold and equal to or better than 10 dB air-bone gap [11].

A target of continuous debate in surgery of stapes fixation is the long-term postsurgical hearing results after stapedectomy and stapedotomy. Table 12.3 shows that the difference in hearing outcome is negligible between the two types of stapes surgeries. The surgical technique is an important aspect of this question. Good hemostasis during surgery helps to avoid application of suction in the oval window niche. This prevents the high-frequency hearing loss.

Not only the hearing improvement and lack of complication and revision surgery which determine the satisfaction of the patient after stapes surgery. The quality of life after stapes surgery is strongly related to postsurgical tinnitus, dizziness, sound distortion, and hearing in noise [16]. A >15 dB improvement in air conduction, postoperatively, significantly improves communication skills, watching TV, and listening to radio [16]. An operation benefit profile [17] establishes the outcome on the basis of the Glasgow hearing-aid benefit profile [18] which is a questionnaire to evaluate listening capabilities in four different situations provided by a hearing aid. Clinically, no significant difference can be found in the literature between the hearing outcome of stapedectomy and stapedotomy in the case of stapes fixation.

Piston diameter is another question which excited the stapes surgeons for many years. Three different sizes were attempted to be used in the clinical practice. These are the 0.4, 0.6, and 0.8 mm diameter pistons. According to a meta-analysis of the literature, the 0.6 mm piston proved to be superior to the 0.4 mm piston both in terms of air-bone gap closure and success rate of the surgery [19–21]. The 0.4 mm fenestra did not prove to be more efficient in the higher frequencies. No apparent differences were found between the hearing outcome of 0.6 mm and 0.8 mm pistons in speech frequencies. The smaller fenestra served with better results in the frequency range of 3–8 kHz [22]. The larger the prosthesis diameter, the better the hearing gain at lower (<1 kHz) frequencies [23–25].

12.2 Vertigo

A persistent vertigo after stapes surgery may occur when the length of the piston is not appropriately chosen. This can be avoided by measuring the distance between the footplate level and the long process of the incus [26]. In general, a 4.75 mm piston length is adequate to provide a good transmission of sound vibrations to the inner ear without stimulating the saccule. A vestibular dysfunction after stapes surgery is a sign of surgical trauma to the membranous labyrinth. A higher incidence of postoperative vertigo has been observed after stapedectomy. This is transient only and does not deteriorate quality of life seriously. Immediate postoperative nystagmus as a transient symptom can be seen in some patients with mild vestibular disorders, e.g., unsteadiness [27, 28]. It does not prolong the hospitalization time. Stapes surgery can be performed as a daycare procedure.

12.3 Tinnitus

Tinnitus of blowing wind character is a typical symptom in stapes fixations. Postoperatively this tinnitus usually disappears. High-frequency tinnitus, however, is resistant against surgery. In a retrospective study, 80 % of patients suffered from preoperative tinnitus. Approx. 60 % of cases postoperatively did not suffer any more from tinnitus [29]. In a prospective study with limited number of participants, the mean preoperative tinnitus discomfort grade was 2.72; at day 1 after surgery, it was 1.29; and after 1 month, it had decreased to 0.96, indicating a significant improvement in the level of tinnitus discomfort (Newman method: grade 1–5). One month after surgery, 82 % of patients had a complete or partial disappearance of tinnitus [30]. In another study, Sparano et al. [31] found that 85 % of patients had improvement in tinnitus grade and 52 % reported about complete resolution of the tinnitus. A separate entity is association of otosclerosis with endolymphatic hydrops as a result of foci around the vestibular aqueduct leading to low-frequency tinnitus and vertigo [32, 33]. Stapedotomy should be preferred in Meniere's disease to avoid disruption of the membranous labyrinth.

12.4 Standards for Evaluation of Postsurgical Functional Benefits in Surgery of Stapes Fixations

1. Lack of major complications.
2. Hearing by air conduction is better than 30 dB threshold at speech frequencies (0.5, 1, 2, 3 kHz) in pure conductive hearing loss or 10 dB or less air-bone gap in mixed hearing loss.
3. Tinnitus is not present as a result of surgery.
4. Disequilibrium is mild and transient in the early postoperative period.

References

1. Karosi T, Csomor P, Tetko M, Liktor B, Szabo LZ, Pytel J, Jori J, Sziklai I. Histopathology of nonotosclerotic stapes fixations. Otol Neurotol. 2009;30:1058–66.
2. Karosi T, Konya J, Petko M, Szabo LZ, Pytel J, Jori J, Sziklai I. Antimeasles immunoglobulin G for serologic diagnosis of otosclerotic hearing loss. Laryngoscope. 2006;116:488–93.

3. Somers T, Vercruysse JP, Zarowski A. Transient depression of inner ear function after stapedectomy: skeeter versus CO_2 laser technique. Adv Otorhinolaryngol. 2007;65:267–72.
4. Wegner I, Kamalski DM, Tange RA, Vincent R, Stegeman I, van der Heijden GJ, Grolman W. Laser versus conventional fenestration in stapedotomy for otosclerosis: a systematic review. Laryngoscope. 2014;124:1687–9.
5. Gerard JM, Serry P, Gersdorff MC. Outcome and lack of prognostic factors in stapes surgery. Otol Neurotol. 2008;29:290–4.
6. De Bruijn AJ, Tange RA, Dreschler WA. Efficacy of evaluation of audiometric results after stapes surgery in otosclerosis. Otolaryngol Head Neck Surg. 2001;124:76 83.
7. Gristwood RE, Venables WN. Effects of fenestra size and piston diameter on the outcome of stapes surgery for clinical otosclerosis. Ann Otol Rhinol Laryngol. 2011;120:363–71.
8. Fish U. Stapedotomy versus stapedectomy. Otol Neurotol. 2009;30:1160–5.
9. Vincent R, Sperling NM, Oates J, Jindal M. Surgical findings and long term hearing results in 3050 stapedotomies for primary otosclerosis. A prospective study with the Otology-Neurotology database. Otol Neurotol. 2006;27:525–47.
10. St. Martin MB, Rubinstein EN, Hirsch BE. High frequency sensorineural hearing loss after stapedectomy. Otol Neurotol. 2008;29:447–52.
11. Sperling NM, Sury K, Gordon J, Cox S. Early postoperative results in stapedectomy. Otolaryngol Head Neck Surg. 2013;149:918–23.
12. Gristwood RE, Venables WN. Analysis of long-term hearing gains after stapes surgery with piston reconstruction for otosclerosis. Ann Otol Rhinol Laryngol. 2013;122:500–10.
13. Antonelli PJ, Gianoli GJ, Lundi LB, et al. Raly post-laser stapedotomy hearing thresholds. Am J Otol. 1988;19:443–6.
14. Hazenberg AJC, Minovi A, Dazert S, Hoppe FF. Predictors of listening capabilities and patient satisfaction after stapes surgery in otosclerosis. Otol Neurotol. 2013;34:220–6.
15. Sennaroğlu L, Unal OF, Sennaroğlu G, Gürsel B, Belgin E. Effect of teflon piston diameter on hearing result after stapedotomy. Otolaryngol Head Neck Surg. 2001;124:279–81.
16. Persson P, Harder H, Magnuson B. Hearing results in otosclerosis surgery after partial stapedectomy, total stapedectomy and stapedotomy. Acta Otolaryngol (Stockh). 1997;117:94–9.
17. Tan FM, Grolman W, Tange RA, Fokkens WJ. Quality of perceived sound after stapedectomy. Otolaryngol Head Neck Surg. 2007;137:443–9.
18. Gatehouse S. Glasgow Hearing Aid Benefit Profile derivation and validation of a client-centred outcome measure for hearing aid services. J Am Acad Audiol. 1999;10:80–103.
19. Cavaliere M, Riccardiello F, Mesolella M, Iengo M. Stapedotomy: functional results with different diameter prosthesis. ORL J Otorhinolaryngol Relat Spec. 2012;74:93–6.
20. Laske RD, Röösli C, Chatzimichalis MV, Sim JH, Huber AM. The influence of prosthesis diameter in stapes surgery: a meta-analysis and systematic review of the literature. Otol Neurotol. 2011;32:520–8.
21. Shabana YK, Ghonim MR, Pedersen CB. Stapedotomy: does prosthesis diameter affect outcome? Clin Otolaryngol Allied Sci. 1999;24:91–4.
22. Domenech J, Carulla M. High frequency audiometric changes after stapedectomy. Scand Audiol Suppl. 1988;30:233–5.
23. Colletti V, Ricci V. Changes in bone conduction threshold during stapedectomy. In: Myers E, editor. New dimensions in otorhinolaryngology – head and neck surgery, vol. 2. Amsterdam: Elsevier; 1985. p. 18–20.
24. Marchese MR, Cianfrone S, Passali GC, Paludetti G. Hearing results after stapedotomy: role of the prosthesis diameter. Audiol Neurotol. 2007;12:221–5.
25. Mair LWS, Laukli E. Air conduction thresholds after myringoplasty and stapes surgery: a conventional and high frequency audiometric comparison. Ann Otol Rhinol Laryngol. 1986;95:327–30.
26. Scierski W, Namysłowski G, Czerwińska G, Lisowska G, Kluczewska E, Bożek P. Postoperative vertigo caused by too long stapes prosthesis – radiological diagnostics. Otolaryngol Pol. 2012;66:363–7.
27. Hirvonen TP, Aalto H. Immediate postoperative nystagmus and vestibular symptoms after stapes surgery. Acta Otolaryngol. 2013;133:842–5.
28. Ozmen AO, Aksoy S, Ozmen S, Saraç S, Sennaroğlu L, Gürsel B. Balance after stapedotomy: analysis of balance with computerized dynamic posturography. Clin Otolaryngol. 2009;34:212–7.
29. Bast F, Mazurek B, Schrom T. Effect of stapedotomy on pre-operative tinnitus and its psychosomatic burden. Auris Nasus Larynx. 2013;40:530–3.
30. Rajati M, Poursadegh M, Bakhshaee M, Abbasi A, Shahabi A. Outcome of stapes surgery for tinnitus recovery in otosclerosis. Int Tinnitus J. 2012;17:42–6.
31. Sparano A, Leonetti JP, Marzo S, Kim H. Effects of stapedectomy on tinnitus in patients with otosclerosis. Int Tinnitus J. 2004;10:73–7.
32. Issa TK, Bahgat MA, Linthicum Jr FH, House HP. The effect of stapedectomy on hearing of patients with otosclerosis and Meniere's disease. Am J Otol. 1983;4:323–6.
33. Yoon TH, Paparella MM, Schachern PA. Otosclerosis involving the vestibular aqueduct and Menière's disease. Otolaryngol Head Neck Surg. 1990;103:107–12.

Index

I. Sziklai (ed.), *Surgery of Stapes Fixations*, DOI 10.1007/978-3-319-28576-4

MIX
Papier aus verantwortungsvollen Quellen
Paper from responsible sources
FSC® C105338

If you have any concerns about our products,
you can contact us on
ProductSafety@springernature.com

In case Publisher is established outside the EU,
the EU authorized representative is:
Springer Nature Customer Service Center GmbH
Europaplatz 3, 69115 Heidelberg, Germany

Printed by Libri Plureos GmbH
in Hamburg, Germany